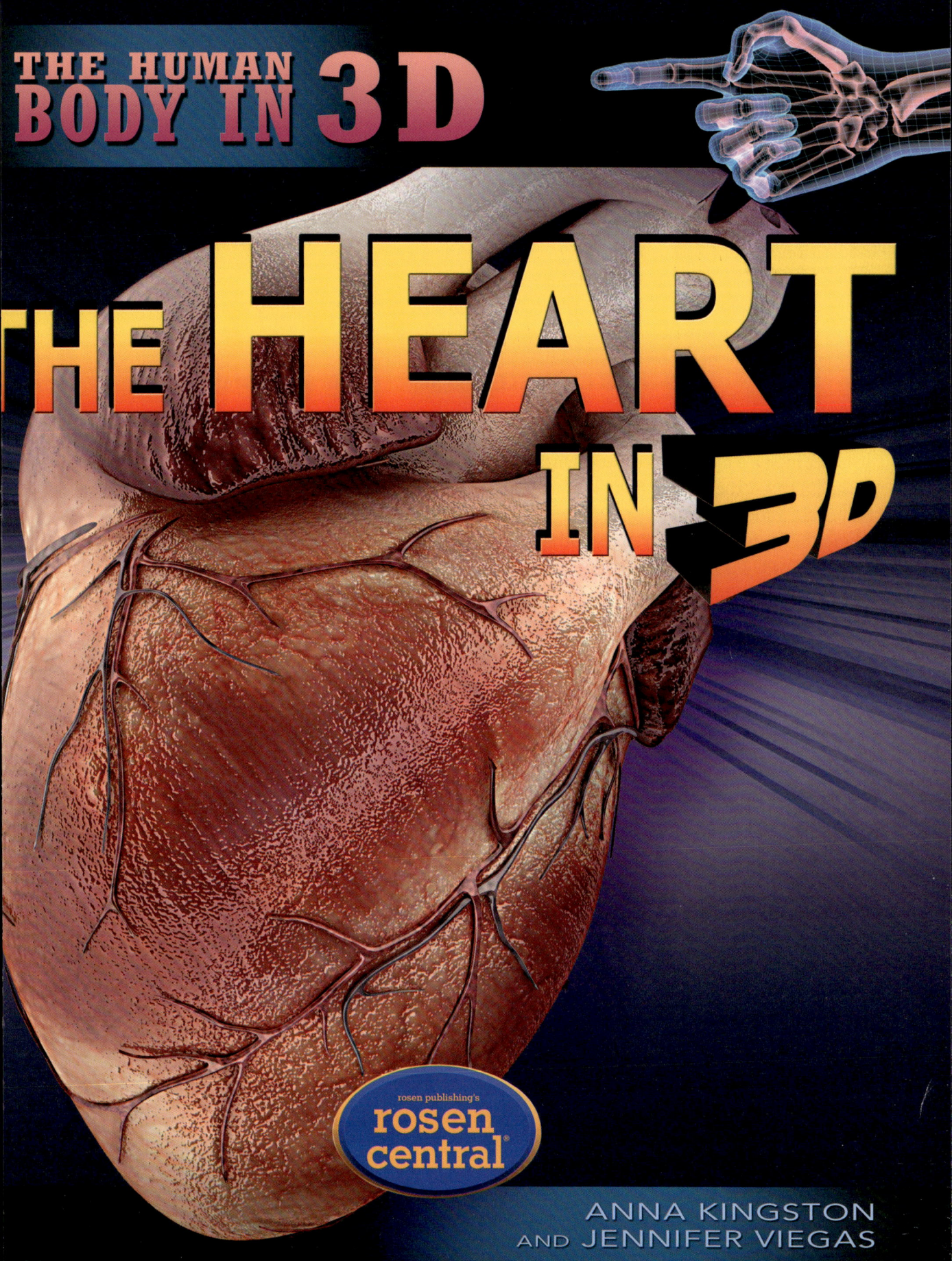

THE HUMAN BODY IN 3D

THE HEART IN 3D

rosen publishing's
rosen central®

ANNA KINGSTON
AND JENNIFER VIEGAS

Published in 2016 by The Rosen Publishing Group, Inc.
29 East 21st Street, New York, NY 10010

Copyright © 2016 by The Rosen Publishing Group, Inc.

First Edition

All rights reserved. No part of this book may be reproduced in any form without permission in writing from the publisher, except by a reviewer.

Library of Congress Cataloging-in-Publication Data

Kingston, Anna.
The heart in 3D/Anna Kingston and Jennifer Viegas.—First edition.
　　pages cm.—(The human body in 3D)
Audience: Grades 5 to 8.
Includes bibliographical references and index.
ISBN 978-1-4994-3597-9 (library bound) — ISBN 978-1-4994-3599-3 (pbk.) — ISBN 978-1-4994-3600-6 (6-pack)
1. Heart—Juvenile literature. 2. Blood—Circulation—Juvenile literature. 3. Cardiovascular system—Juvenile literature. I. Viegas, Jennifer. II. Title.
QP111.6.K56 2016
612.1'7—dc23

2015000195

Manufactured in the United States of America

CONTENTS

INTRODUCTION 4

CHAPTER ONE
THE HUMAN HEART 9

CHAPTER TWO
BLOOD 18

CHAPTER THREE
MOVING THROUGH THE SYSTEM 28

CHAPTER FOUR
THE KIDNEYS 40

GLOSSARY 52

FOR MORE INFORMATION 55

FOR FURTHER READING 59

INDEX 61

INTRODUCTION

People often use the word "heart" to describe the innermost, most essential part of something. It makes sense, then, that the human heart is among the most essential organs in the body. The heart pumps blood throughout the body, propelling it through a system of blood vessels. This blood, which the heart circulates in an endless loop, has several important jobs. It distributes oxygen and nutrients to cells throughout the body. The body's cells need these to continue to do their own individual jobs. Blood also carries away the waste that cells throughout the body produce. It releases carbon dioxide into the lungs, from which we breathe it out. The kidneys filter out other kinds of wastes. Together, the organs and tissues that transport blood around the body make up the cardiovascular system.

The heart is a truly amazing organ. In a single day, it pumps blood through more than 60,000 miles (96,560

The average human body has about 5.8 quarts (5.5 liters) of blood. The heart pumps blood throughout the body, while the kidneys filter waste out of blood.

INTRODUCTION

kilometers) of vessels. That is like traveling from California to New York more than twenty times in twenty-four hours! Blood is itself a pretty incredible substance. There are three kinds of blood cells, each important for a different reason. Red blood cells absorb and transport oxygen. White blood cells keep us healthy by fighting off infections. Platelets allow blood to clot, which repairs blood vessels and keeps us from losing too much blood if we get cut or otherwise injured. The circulation of blood throughout the body helps maintain a constant temperature and pH (pH is a measure of the acidity or basicity of a substance) throughout the body.

Unfortunately, there are a number of things that can go wrong with the cardiovascular system. Some are congenital, or things people are born with. Others result from illness, injury, or unhealthy habits. Problems with the heart's rhythm are called arrhythmias. Cardiomyopathy is the enlargement of the heart or the thickening of its muscle. When the valves—which allow the flow of blood through the different parts of the heart—do not function properly, they can cause a heart murmur. Atherosclerosis, often known as heart disease, is the buildup and hardening of plaque—a waxy substance made primarily of cholesterol—in the blood vessels. It can lead to angina, or chest pain. A heart attack happens when the flow of blood to the heart is blocked. If the flow of blood to the brain is blocked, a stroke occurs. Heart failure occurs when the heart's muscle is no longer able to keep pumping blood at the rate it should.

While the problems that affect the heart and rest of the cardiovascular system are myriad and serious, there are steps you can take to maintain you heart health. For one, stick to a diet

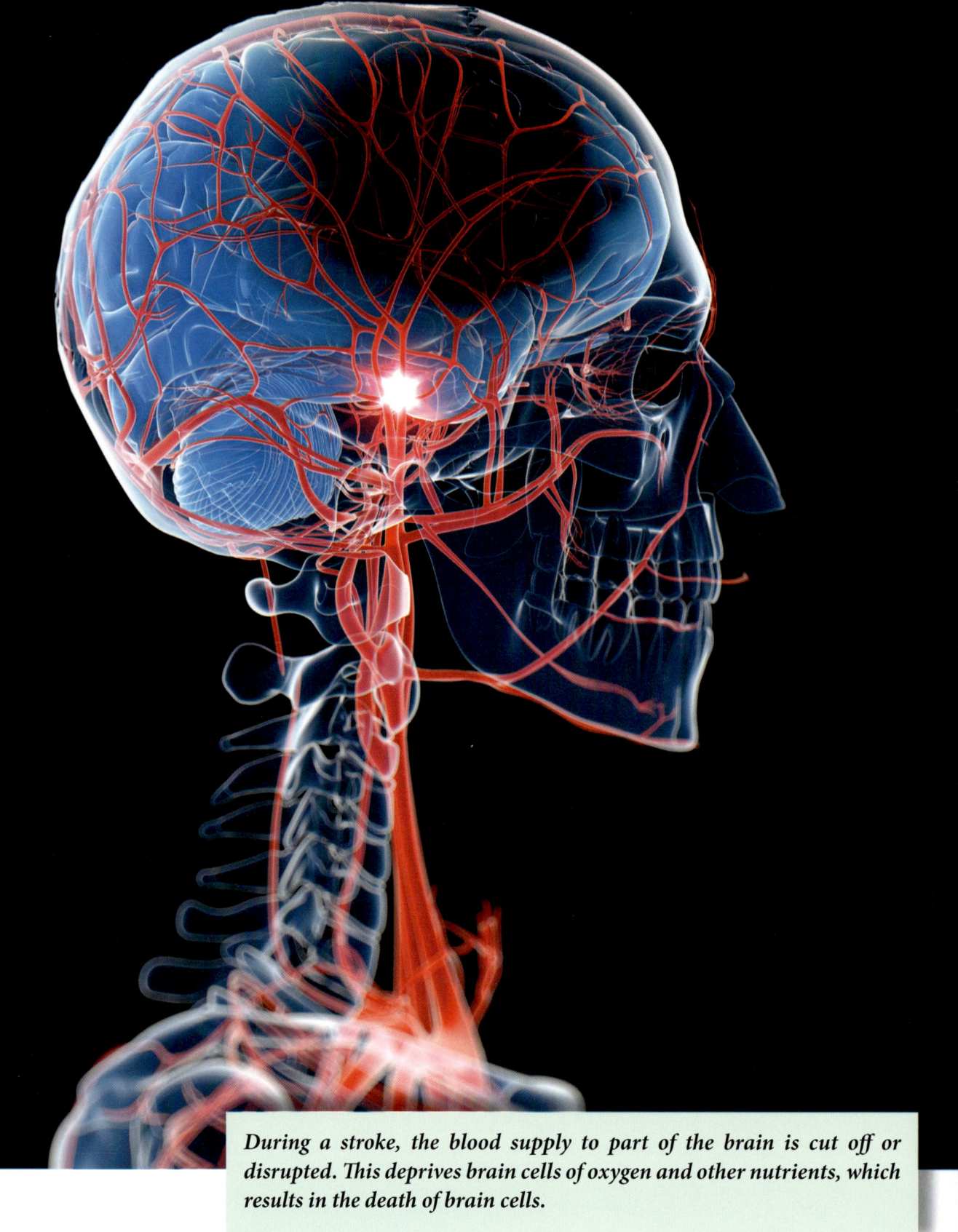

During a stroke, the blood supply to part of the brain is cut off or disrupted. This deprives brain cells of oxygen and other nutrients, which results in the death of brain cells.

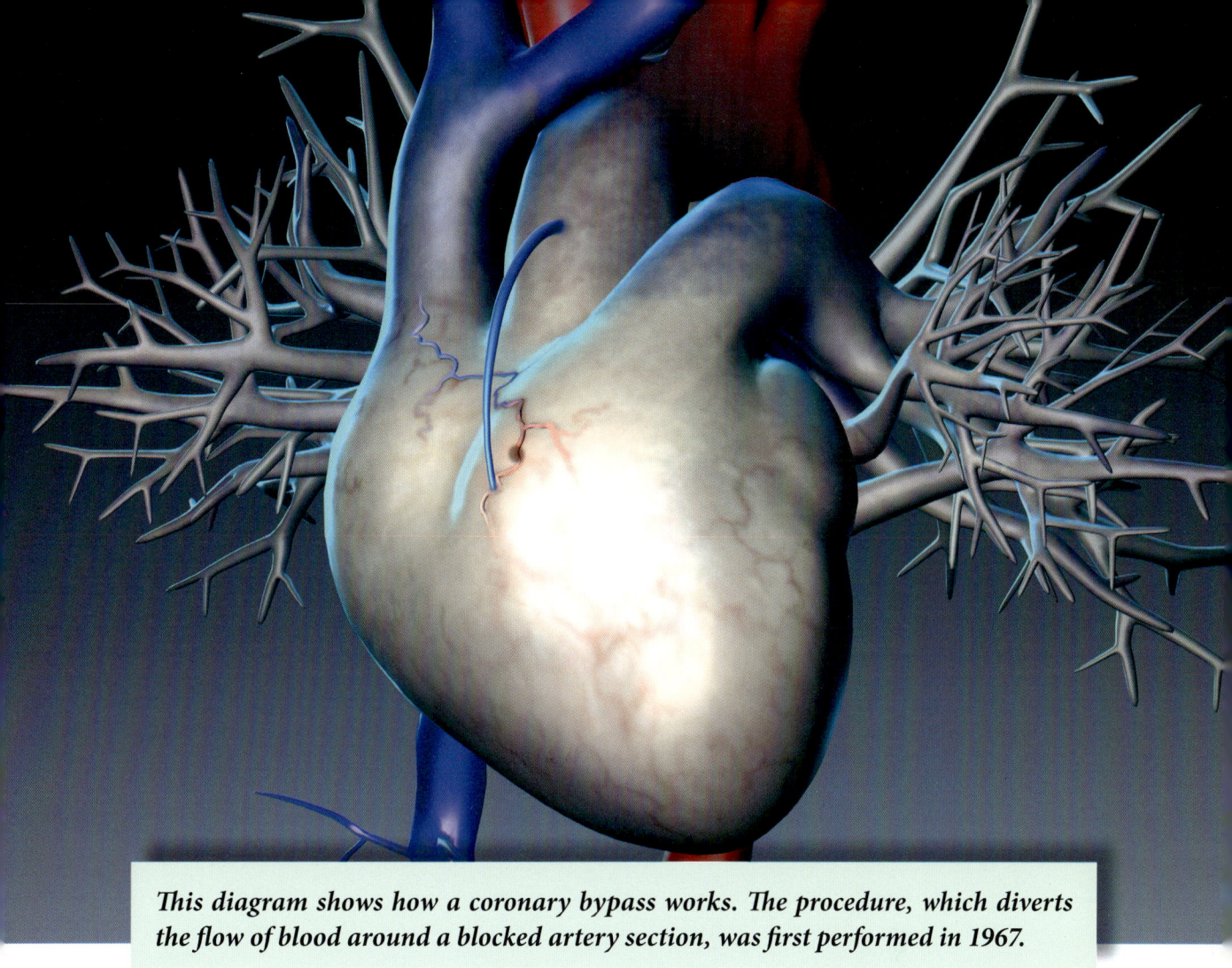

This diagram shows how a coronary bypass works. The procedure, which diverts the flow of blood around a blocked artery section, was first performed in 1967.

that is low in fat, salt, sugar, and cholesterol. These not only cause atherosclerosis but also contribute to conditions such as high blood pressure, high cholesterol, and diabetes (all of which are, in their turn, risk factors for heart disease). Don't smoke and try to avoid high-stress situations. Getting regular exercise is good for your heart. So is good hygiene.

Modern technology has also provided us with some amazing ways to treat cardiovascular problems. Coronary bypass surgery introduces a new path through which blood can flow from one part of the heart to another, bypassing an artery that has become blocked. In an angioplasty, a thin tube is inserted into a blocked blood vessel and then a balloon or other device is used to unblock the vessel by pushing the plaque against the vessel walls. Small devices called pacemakers can be inserted into the heart to send out electrical impulses that correct the heart's rhythm. In a heart transplant surgery, a damaged heart is removed and replaced by a healthy heart, which comes from the body of someone who has recently died. Doctors go to such measures to treat heart problems because the heart is so essential. After all, checking if someone has a heartbeat is one of the classic ways to figure out if that person is still alive.

CHAPTER ONE

THE HUMAN HEART

An actual human heart bears little resemblance to the iconic heart shape you see everywhere on Valentine's Day. Instead, it is a hollow, fist-shaped ball of muscle with tubes to receive and eject blood. The heart weighs approximately 12 ounces (340 grams), which is about the same as one sneaker. It is located in the middle of the chest area, or thorax, just left of center. For protection, the ribs and breastbone form a sturdy cage around the heart and lungs. A thick sac, called the pericardium, helps to hold the heart in place within the bony cage.

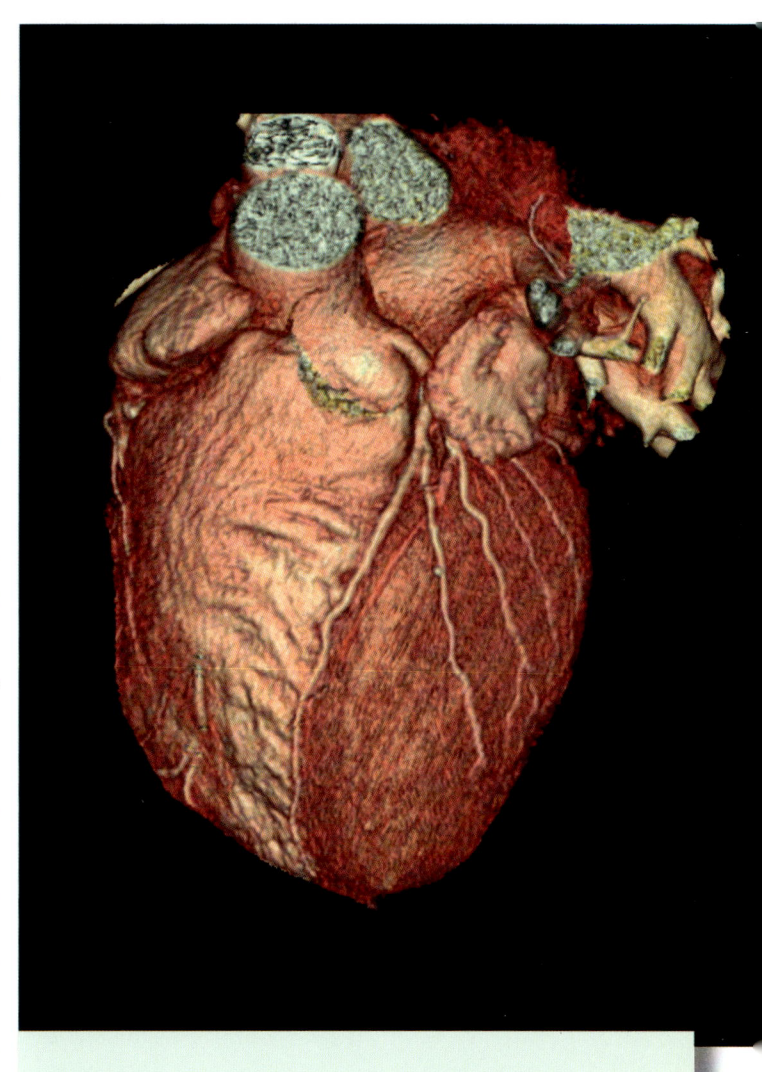

This CT scan shows what a normal heart looks like. The CT (short for computed tomography) process uses X-ray technology to produce 3D images.

THE HEART IN 3D

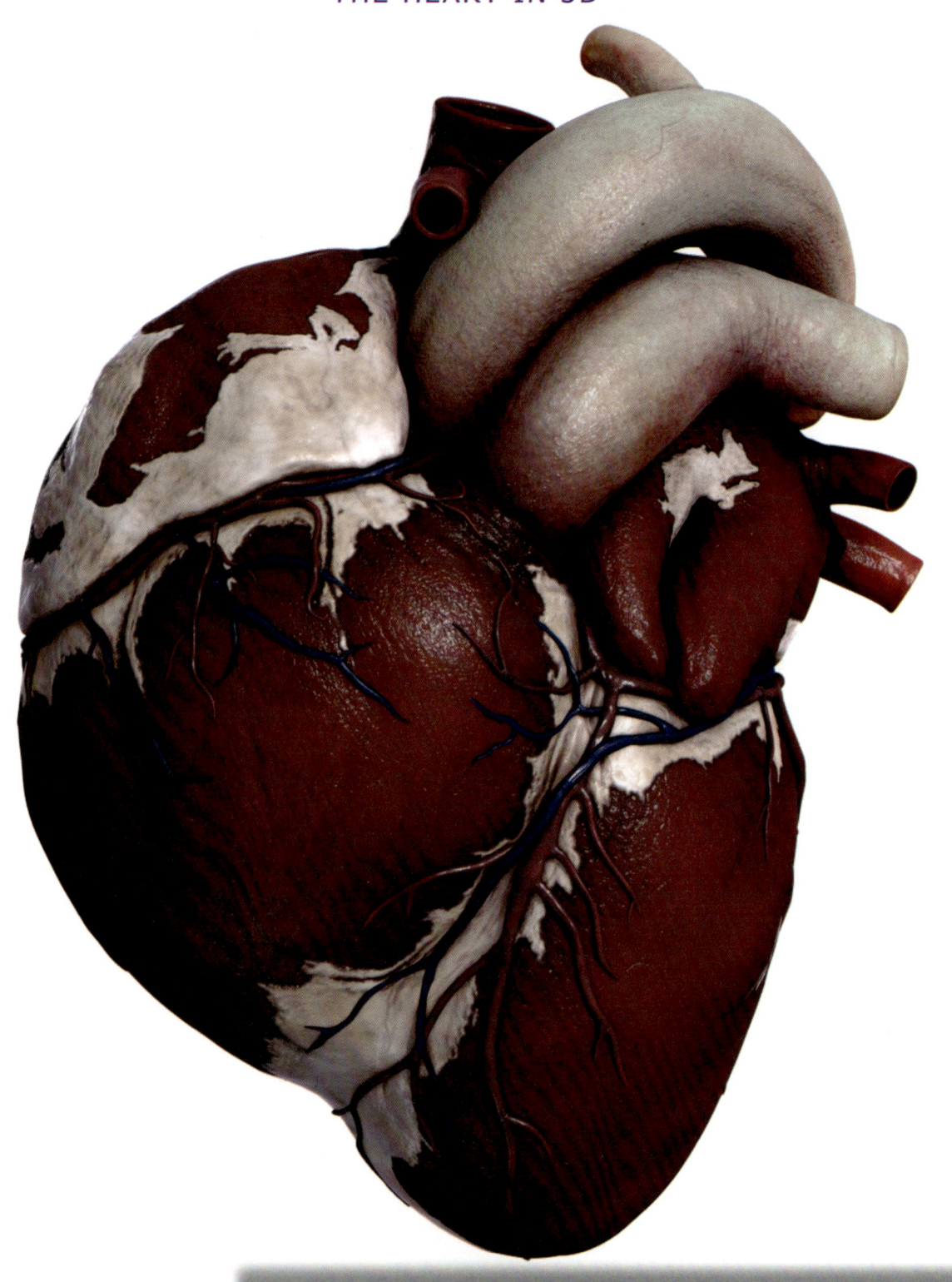

A layer of tissue called the epicardium covers the myocardium, while a layer of tissue called the endocardium makes up the inner layer of the heart.

A MAJOR MUSCLE

Somewhat resembling roots from a plant, arteries and veins are attached to the heart's surface. They supply food and oxygen, which fuel the heart's nonstop pumping action. Each of these arteries and veins has a name that usually refers to its location on the outside of the heart. The thick-stranded sections near the top portion of the heart are the right coronary artery and the left coronary artery.

"Coronary" comes from the Latin word *corona*, meaning crown, as the ancient Romans highly valued the heart. Many words associated with parts of the body derive from Latin or Greek because their speakers were among the first to study and document human anatomy, or body structure. The word "anatomy" itself actually comes from a Greek phrase meaning "to cut up," as early scientists, like surgeons, had to cut through the skin to find out what was inside the body.

The thick coronary arteries taper off into smaller branches that go directly into the heart. Slightly thinner veins run next to the arteries, with the great cardiac vein going in a top to bottom horizontal direction and the anterior cardiac vein curving around the bottom section of the heart.

The heart itself is constructed of a special muscle called the myocardium, or cardiac muscle. It is very fibrous, like tough strands of rope strung together. The cells that make up the cardiac muscle receive the food and oxygen provided by the coronary arteries.

THE HEART IN 3D

The heart muscle cells work involuntarily, meaning that they work on their own without your having to move them consciously. This is an amazing feature of the heart. Most other muscles require a direct command from the brain. For example, a person must decide whether or not to raise an arm, leg, or hand. The heart, however, beats on its own even when a person is sleeping or resting. Each heartbeat from a resting person sends $1/3$ pint (158 milliliters) of blood, equivalent to about half the contents of a can of soda, throughout the body.

The objects that look like tubes coming out of the heart are large arteries and veins. Arteries move blood away from the heart, while veins bring blood to the heart. The large faucet-like object at the top of the heart with three tubular appendages makes up the aorta. Similar to a high-pressure

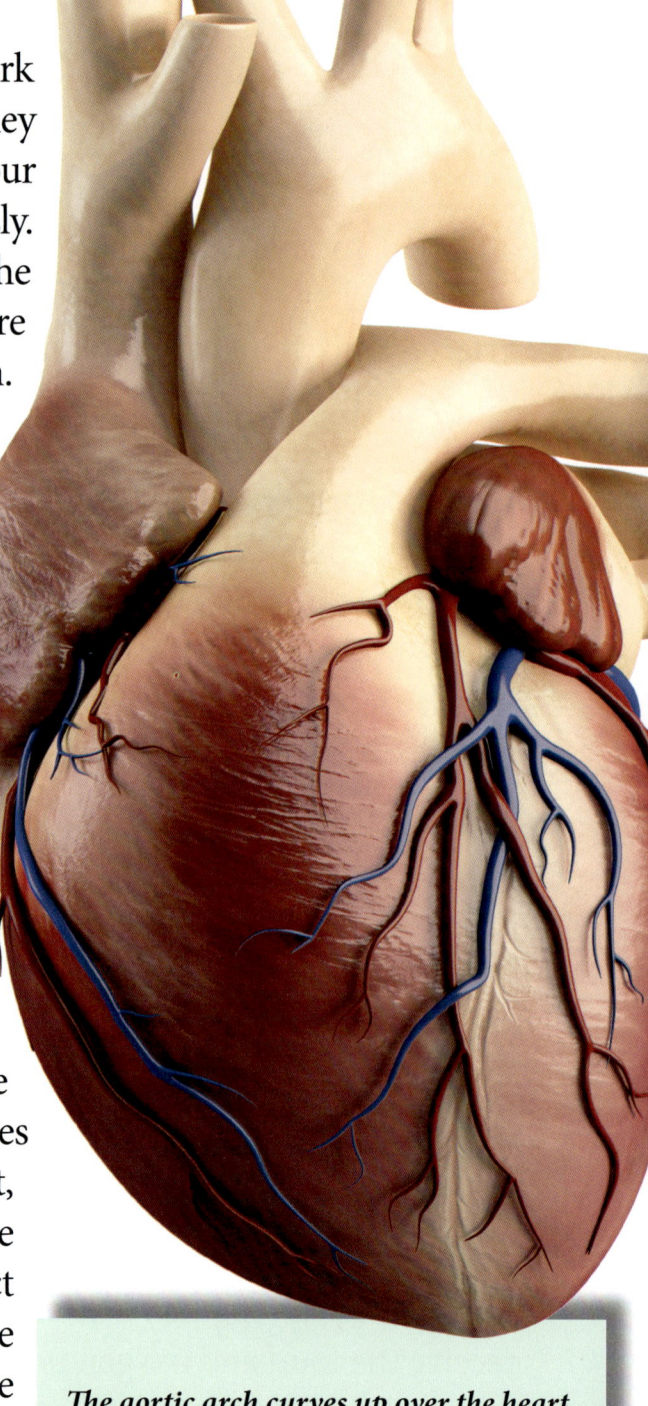

The aortic arch curves up over the heart. The brachiocephalic artery, left carotid artery, and left subclavian artery branch out from it. You can see the vena cava to the arch's left here.

water faucet, the aorta shoots blood out of the heart so that it can travel throughout the entire body. Amazingly, blood coming through the aorta travels at a pressure high enough to send water six feet (1.8 meters) in the air.

The large tube underneath the aorta is called the pulmonary artery. It carries blood to the lungs so that the blood can receive oxygen. Liquids like blood can actually hold gas. Think of soda, which gets its fizz from the gas carbon dioxide. Blood retains oxygen and distributes it to other parts of the body. The two connected tubes sticking out from under the pulmonary artery form the pulmonary vein, which carries blood from the lungs to the heart.

VALVES AND CHAMBERS

A cross-section view of the heart reveals that it actually consists of two pumps joined together. There is a pump on the left side and a pump on the right side. Each has a small upper chamber, or enclosed space, known as the atrium. Below the atrium is a doughnut-shaped disk that functions as a valve. The left disk is called the tricuspid valve, while the one on the right is called the mitral valve. The valves open and close, controlling blood flow into the bottom chambers, known as ventricles. The left ventricle is very strong, much stronger than the right ventricle. That is because it is responsible for pumping blood to every part of the body, from the head to the tips of the toes. Extending from the valves are jellyfish-like tendrils. Their scientific name is chordae tendineae. These help to control the valves and

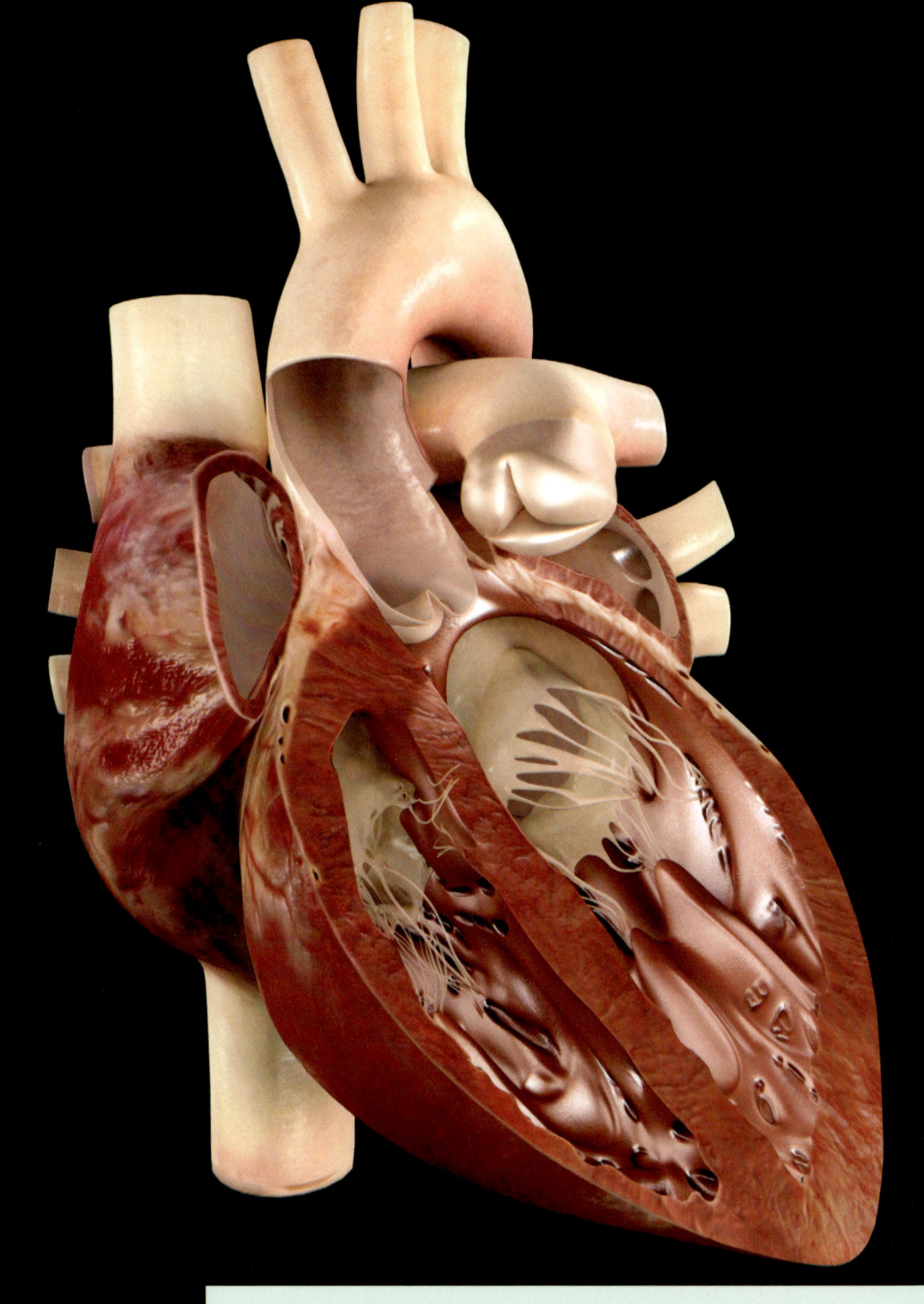

The right side of the heart—consisting of the right ventricle and right atrium—deals with oxygen-poor blood. Oxygen-rich blood flows through the heart's left ventricle and atrium.

prevent blood from flowing backward. A third valve, located in the top center of the heart, does not have the tendril extensions. It is called the tricuspid valve, and it controls blood flow from the right ventricle to the lungs through the pulmonary artery. A fourth valve, called the aortic valve, prevents blood from flowing backward into the left ventricle.

THE HEART'S RHYTHM

When a doctor listens to a patient's heartbeat, the doctor is really listening to the valves shutting. A normal heartbeat sounds something like "ba-bump" or, as doctors often say, "lubb-dupp." The "lubb" sound is longer and louder than the "dupp" noise.

WHAT'S YOUR HEARTRATE?

Heart pulse rates can vary, even during rest periods. In humans, age determines how fast a heart beats. Ten-year-olds have hearts that, on average, beat from eighty to ninety times per minute, while adults have a pulse rate of between sixty and eighty beats per minute.

Size affects heart rates, with larger animals like humans having fewer beats per minute than smaller creatures. A tiny mouse, for example, has a very fast heart rate at over five hundred beats per minute. The heavy, muscular heart of a huge elephant, in contrast, beats only twenty to thirty times per minute.

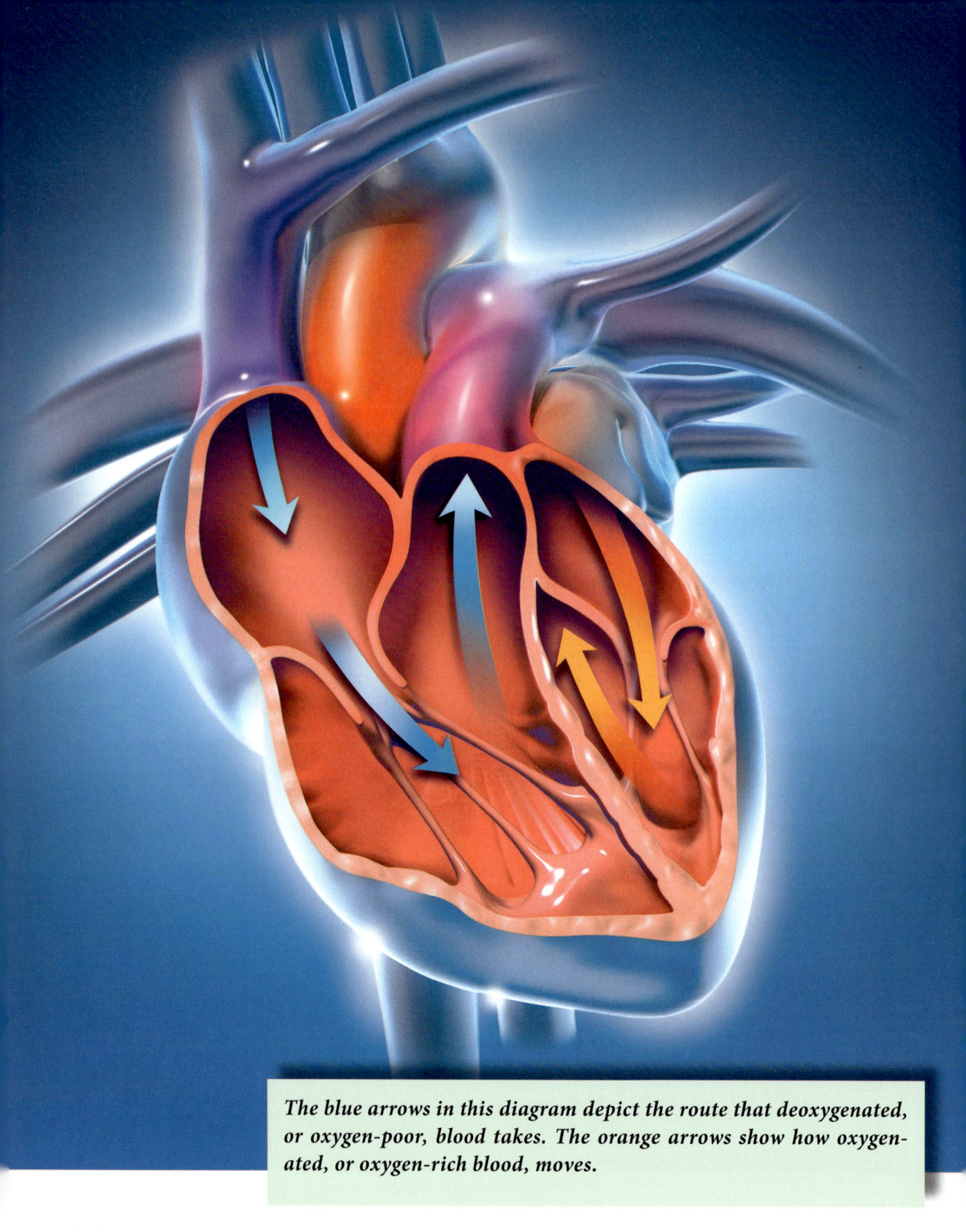

The blue arrows in this diagram depict the route that deoxygenated, or oxygen-poor, blood takes. The orange arrows show how oxygenated, or oxygen-rich blood, moves.

16

Each heartbeat can be divided into three basic stages. First, the right atrium fills with low-oxygen blood from the body and the left atrium fills with high-oxygen blood that has just entered the heart from its trip to the lungs. Second, the muscles of the heart gently squeeze blood through the right and left valves into the ventricles. The ventricles, now full with blood, bulge out.

During the third and final phase, the ventricles contract, or shrink in size. Low-oxygen blood in the right ventricle flows into the lungs. Like a car that is low on fuel, this blood needs energizing. The high-oxygen blood from the left ventricle, on the other hand, is like a car full of gasoline. It is ready for the big journey throughout the body. The aortic valve opens, and the high-oxygen blood in the left ventricle gushes through the aorta with incredible force.

It is amazing to consider that this process occurs every second of every day. During the lifetime of most individuals, the heart will beat over two thousand million times without stopping to rest. There are fuel pumps in sleek cars and pumps that are used to fill the tires of high tech bikes, but nothing surpasses the human pump—the heart—for strength and durability.

CHAPTER TWO

BLOOD

Most individuals see blood only at the doctor's office, while watching a horror movie, or after sustaining a cut or scrape. Blood, however, is always moving around in the body, from the day a person is born until death. This miracle fluid is essential to human life. Pumped by the heart into the arteries, blood delivers oxygen, food, and other essential things to the body.

A LIQUID MIXTURE

Blood is not a simple liquid, like water, but is more like a nourishing smoothie made up of several different ingredients. Blood, as the saying goes, is thicker than water. In fact, it contains millions of individual cells. It is actually considered to be a liquid tissue. Each person has a lot of blood. For an idea of how much, think of it in terms of soft drink cans. A female adolescent has between twelve to fifteen cans worth of blood. A male, depending on size, has slightly more, with between fifteen and eighteen soda cans worth of blood. That

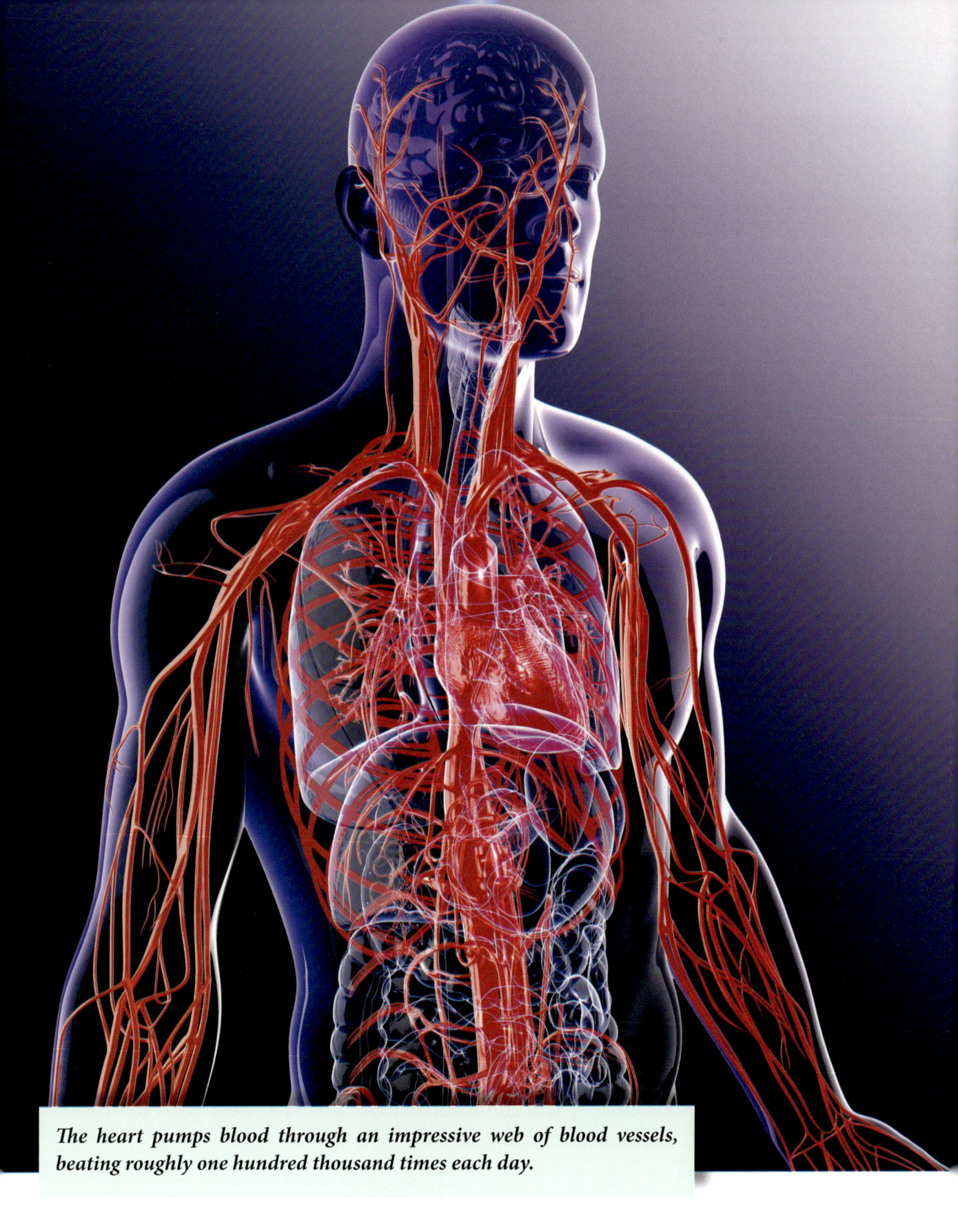

The heart pumps blood through an impressive web of blood vessels, beating roughly one hundred thousand times each day.

is equivalent to three six packs! Imagine drinking that much soda in one day.

To the naked eye, blood looks like a thick, red liquid. Medical specialists can put a vial of blood in a contraption called a centrifuge, which spins things around extremely fast. After spinning in a centrifuge, blood separates into its four basic components: water, plasma, red blood cells, and white blood cells. Water is the lightest of the group, and it makes up about 50 percent of all blood. Plasma is the second lightest, followed by white blood cells and the heavier red blood cells. In just a pinhead-sized drop of blood there are fivew million red blood cells and ten thousand white cells.

GOING WITH THE FLOW

When separated from blood, plasma looks like a pale yellow liquid. Its main function is to carry sugars, fats, and other nutrients throughout the body. One of the primary substances carried by plasma is iron. Iron helps to form a blood protein called hemoglobin, which helps to bring oxygen to cells. Without enough iron, people can develop anemia, a health problem that often requires taking iron pills. That is one reason why it is important to eat foods high in iron, such as leafy green vegetables, dates, and raisins. Plasma also carries hormones, which serve as chemical messengers. Hormones control growth, moods, and lots of other things.

Plasma further contains two types of protein: albumin and globulin. Produced by the liver, albumin helps to monitor blood

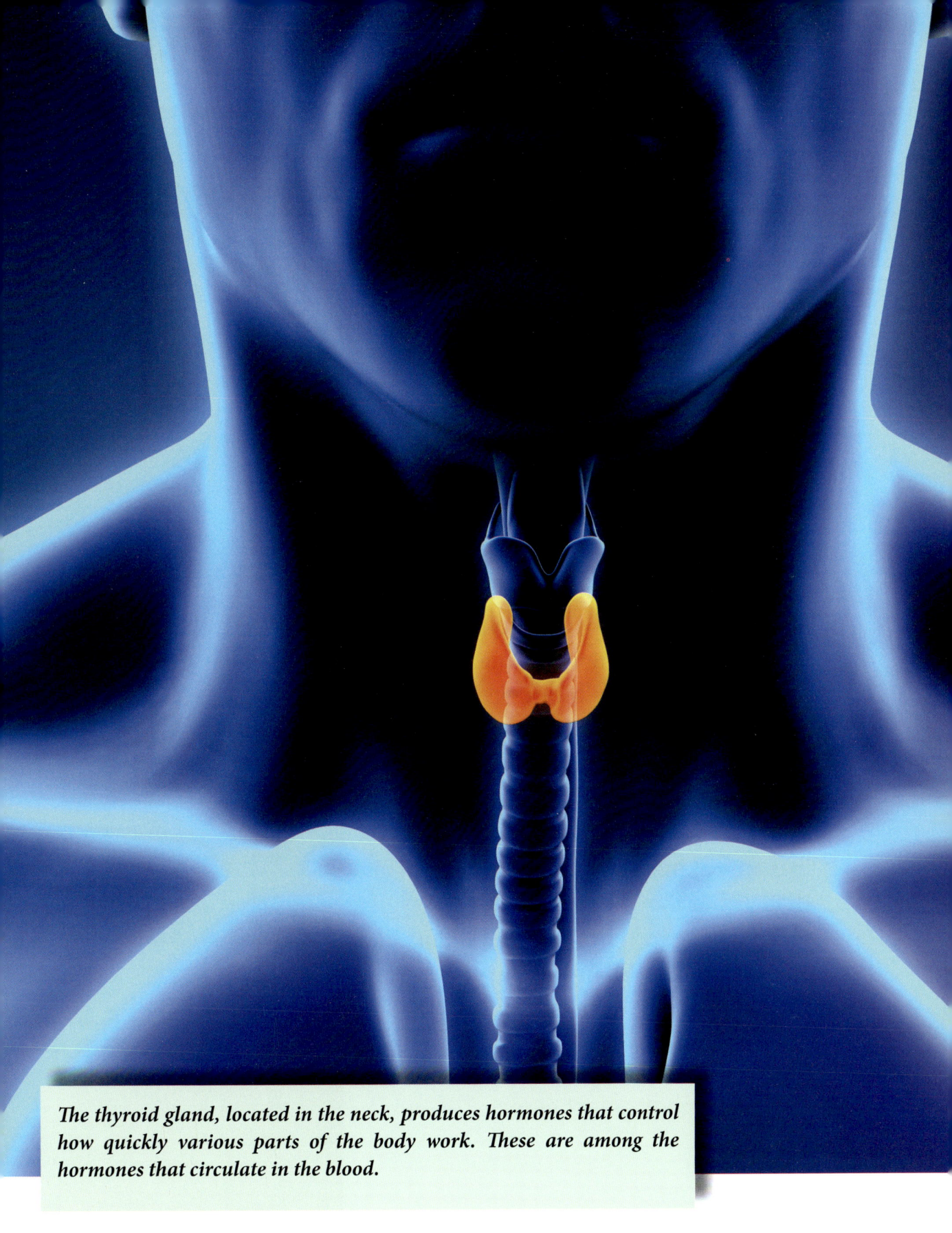

The thyroid gland, located in the neck, produces hormones that control how quickly various parts of the body work. These are among the hormones that circulate in the blood.

flow. It essentially acts like liquid sponge that controls blood and water levels in the body. Without it, the body would have the consistency of jelly due to too much water being absorbed by cells. Globulin helps to fight infection.

CARRYING OXYGEN

Red blood cells look like tiny doughnuts without holes. They are red because this color is produced when their hemoglobin protein combines with oxygen in the lungs. Each day, the body manufactures three million red blood cells in the spongy inner tissue of bone known as marrow. The same number of red blood cells die each day, so the new ones serve as their replacements. Red blood cells live approximately four months. During that time they help to carry oxygen to cells within the body and then, like garbage trucks, fill up with excess wastes that the body does not need, such as the gas carbon dioxide. Carbon dioxide is dumped into the lungs, where a person can exhale and get rid of it.

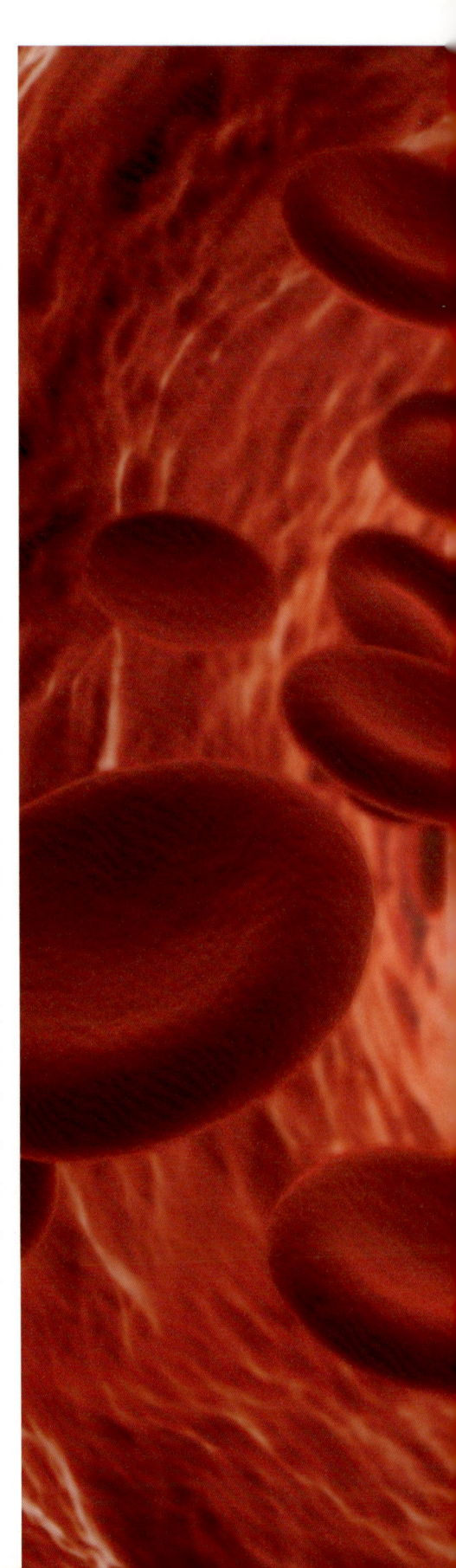

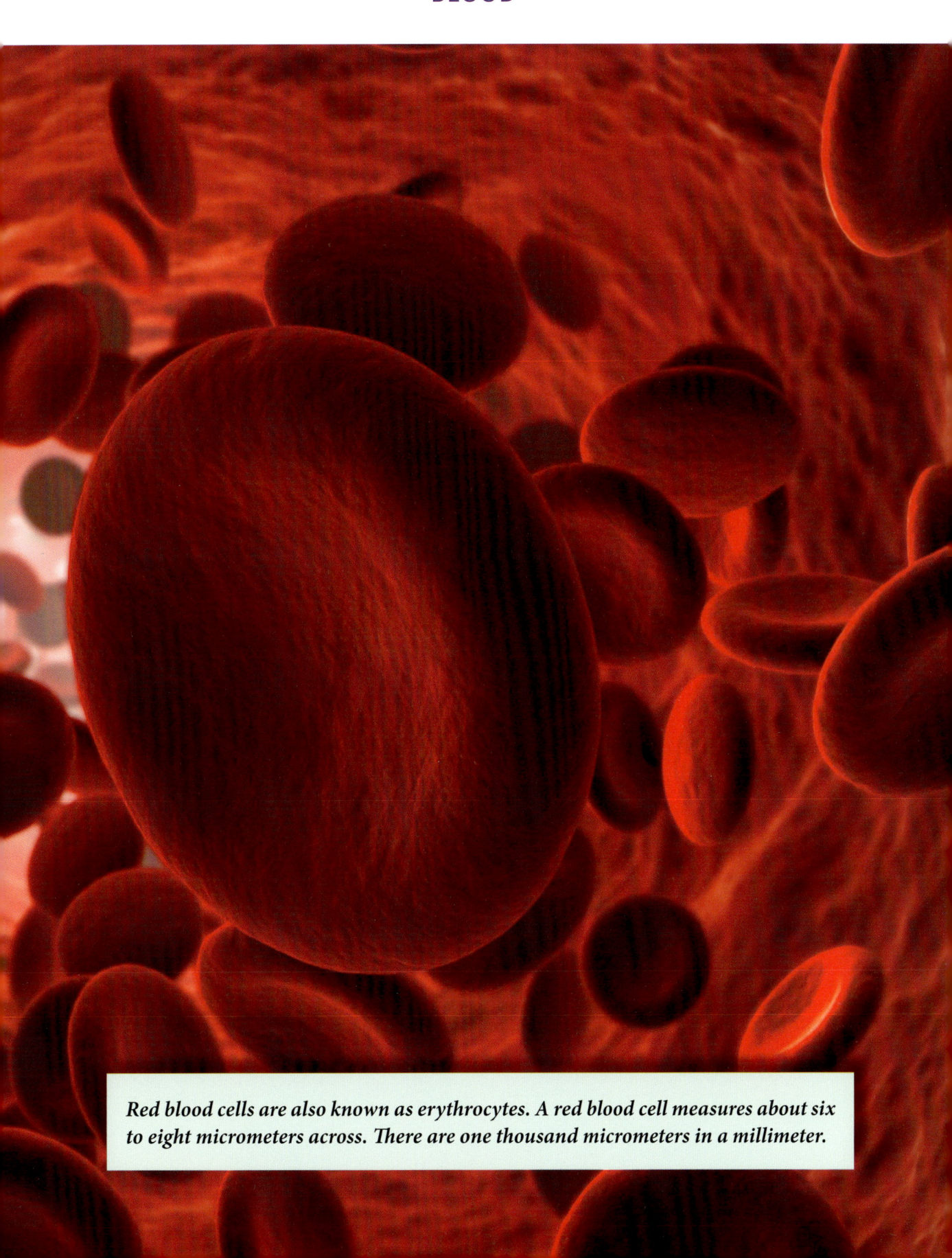

BLOOD

Red blood cells are also known as erythrocytes. A red blood cell measures about six to eight micrometers across. There are one thousand micrometers in a millimeter.

WHAT'S YOUR TYPE?

Like hair color, everyone has his or her own blood type. There are four types: A, B, AB, and O. The letters "A" and "B" refer to special proteins that the body makes, called antigens, which stimulate the body to create germ fighters. Type AB means that a person makes both A and B antigens. Type O blood does not have antigens, but it still possesses antibodies—the germ warriors.

It is important for people to know their blood type before receiving blood from an outside source through a transfusion because certain antigens and antibodies clash and hurt each other.

FIGHTING OFF INFECTION

White blood cells are extremely important for maintaining good health because they fight germs and bacteria. About twice the size of a red blood cell, a white blood cell literally attacks bacteria, eats it up, and destroys it. When a person's nose runs, the mucus is mostly made out of germs and dead white blood cells, which live for only about two weeks. Bone marrow and other parts of the body are constantly making these protective cells.

There are several types of white blood cells. One group falls into a category called lymphocytes, which come from sections of the body called lymph nodes. A person who has an infection might even be able to feel his or her lymph nodes

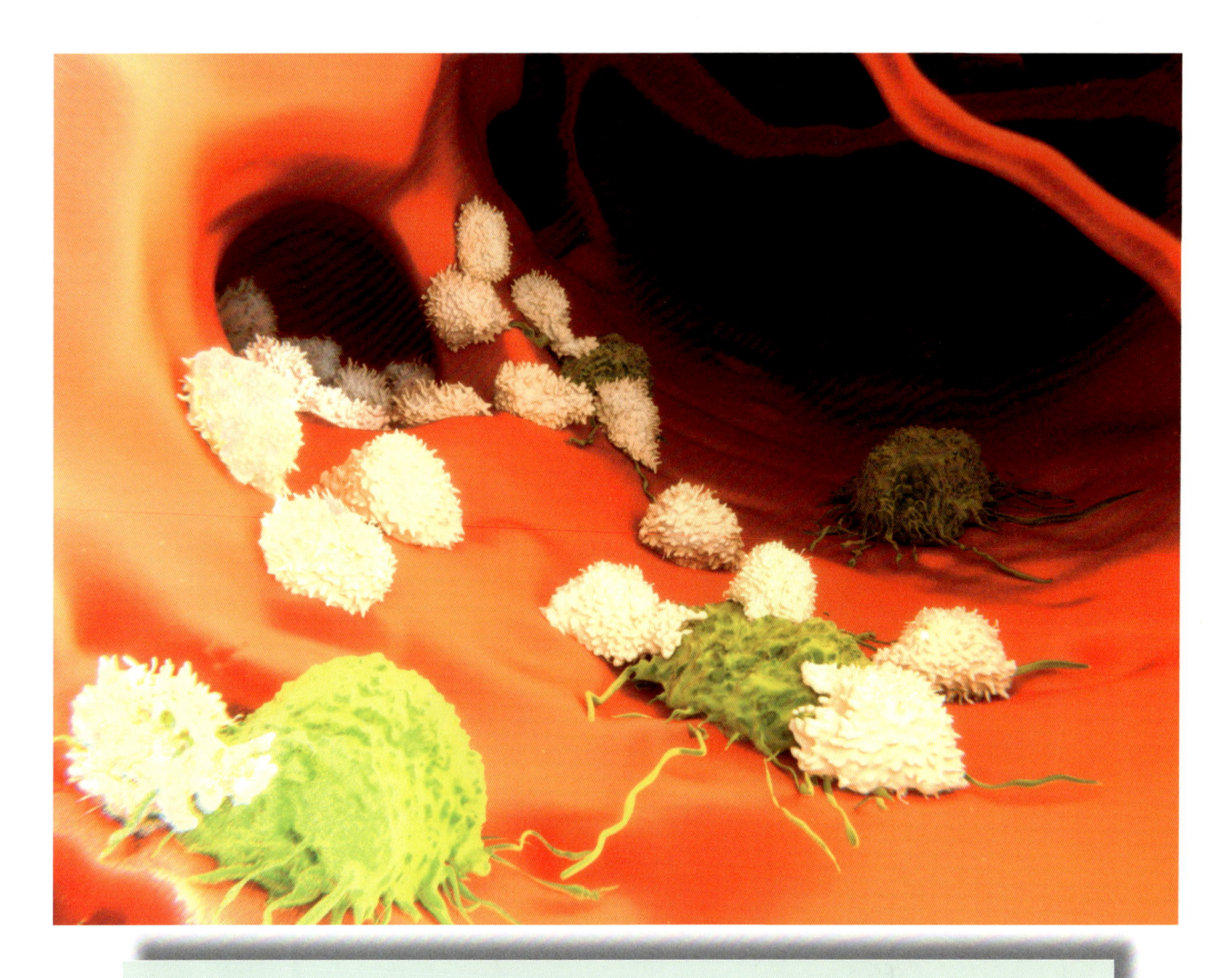

This illustration shows T cells attacking cancer cells. Patients who are sick have high T cell counts because the body makes more of these cells to combat infection.

in the neck because they become swollen with many white blood cell "soldiers" that have tried to fight off the virus. There are two types of lymphocytes: B cells and T cells. B cells make antibodies, or germ fighters, while T cells attack germs and regularly check cells within the body for dangerous chemicals and foreign substances. Doctors often monitor T cell counts in people with serious illnesses, such as cancer or AIDS.

THE HEART IN 3D

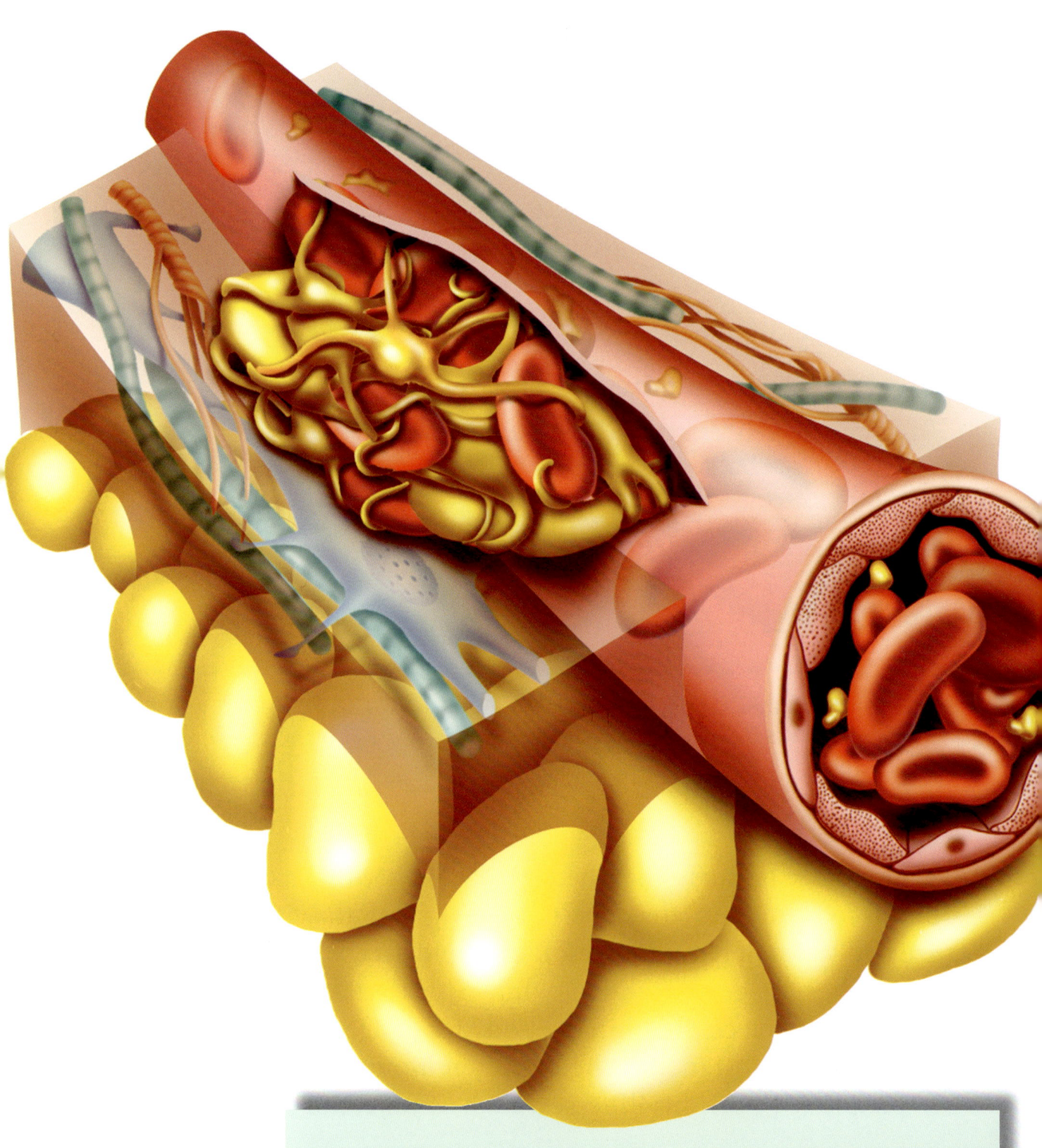

This diagram shows the process of cicatrization, as the formation of a scar on a wound is known.

CLOTTING

Blood also contains platelets, which are distributed throughout its liquid mass. When the skin is cut, blood leaks out of the body because it is under pressure, similar to having juice run out of a sliced orange. Like a kind of super glue, platelets clump together at the site of a wound to prevent too much blood from leaking out and to promote healing. They then develop into a sticky protein called fibrin that nets together to block blood's escape. Chemical reactions make the resulting clot turn hard and solid. When dry, the clot becomes a scab that eventually falls off.

CHAPTER THREE

MOVING THROUGH THE SYSTEM

One way to picture the cardiovascular system is as an intricate network of roads for blood. Blood vessels are laid out like freeways throughout the body. Small arteries and veins are similar to back roads. They lead to deep body tissues and hard-to-reach spots. Major veins and arteries are more like major highways. They carry blood across larger areas and to organs in the body.

Veins and arteries run through every part of the body. Diagrams mapping out these blood vessels appear to show tree-like objects in the chest cavity, with roots snaking out to other areas. The structures resembling trees are actually arteries and veins clustered around major parts of the body, such as the lungs and liver, which affect the contents of blood.

Think of arteries like mail carriers. They deliver essential items, in this case nutrients and oxygen, to cells. Veins, on the other hand, function similar to recycling trucks. They pick up

MOVING THROUGH THE SYSTEM

low-oxygen blood that has already given up its nutrients and return it to the heart and lungs for an energizing refill. The only exception to this is the pulmonary vein, which transports oxygen-rich blood from the lungs to the heart. The basic point to keep in mind is that arteries take blood away from the heart while veins bring blood to the heart.

MOVING AWAY FROM THE HEART

Arteries and veins have different structures suited to the jobs they perform. Since arteries carry blood away from the heart, they need to be thick and sturdy. A cross section of an artery reveals that it is hollow inside. The hollow center, where the blood flows

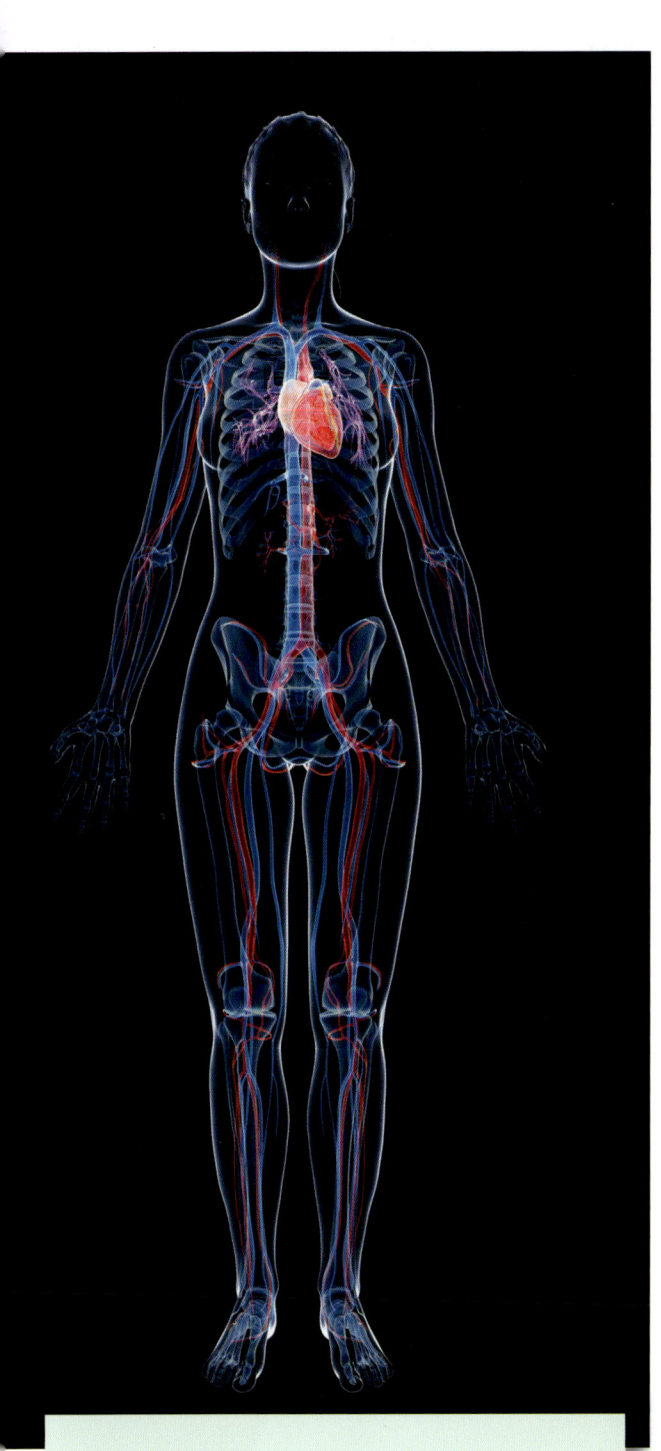

This drawing of a woman's cardiovascular system shows her arteries in red and her veins in blue. Her heart is also red in the image.

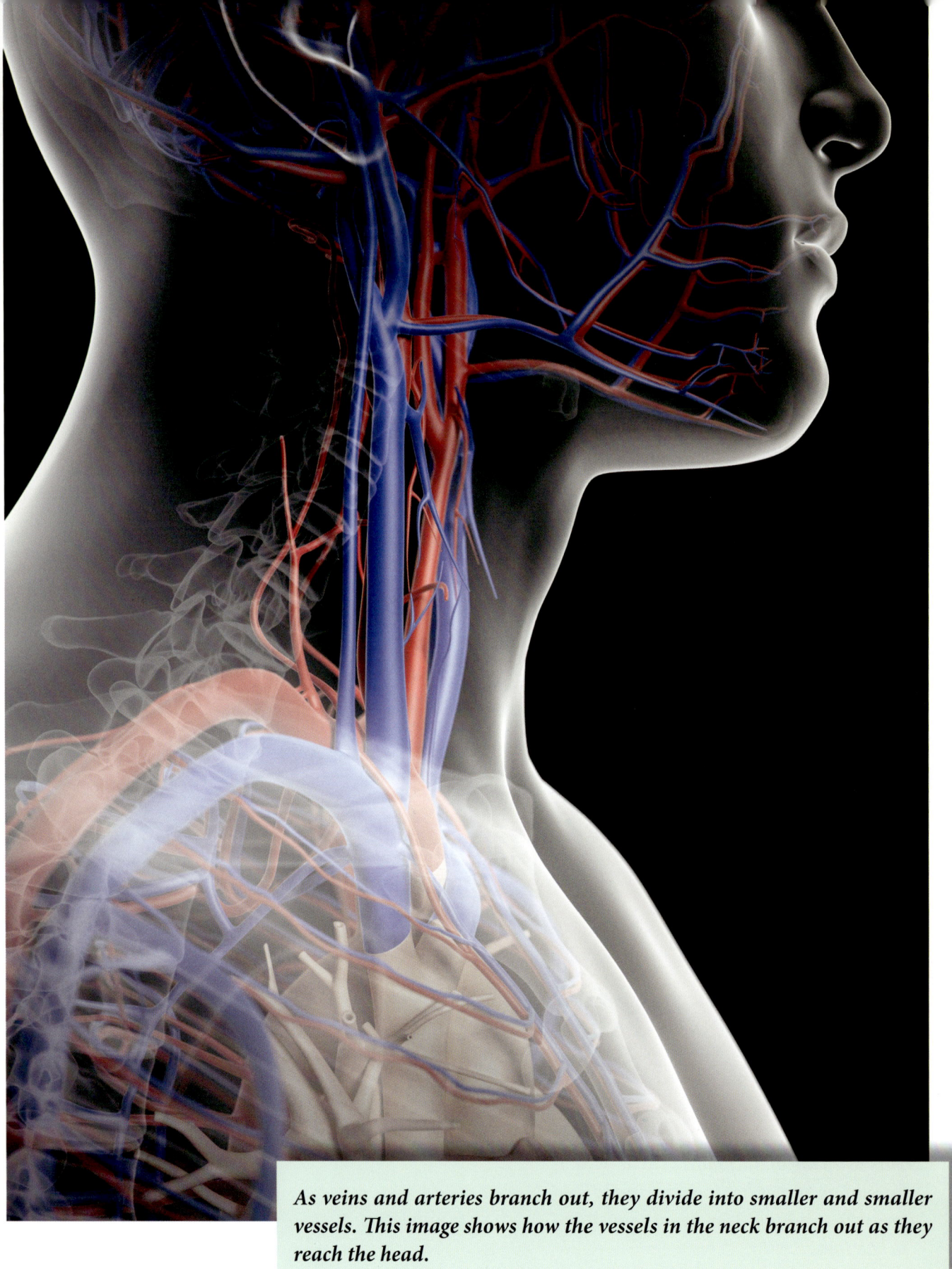

As veins and arteries branch out, they divide into smaller and smaller vessels. This image shows how the vessels in the neck branch out as they reach the head.

through, is called the lumen. The walls of arteries are dense, elastic, and muscular, sort of like a living garden hose that can move to accommodate its contents, yet remain springy enough to flex like a rubber band.

Large arteries are about as wide as a thumb. The biggest artery of all is the aorta, which emerges directly out of the left side of the heart. It is about 1 inch (2.5 centimeters) wide. This amazing artery handles blood pumped at high force with each heartbeat. Its rubbery walls help to ensure that it does not burst under all of the pressure.

Small arteries are called arterioles. Because they are not located as close to the heart, their job is less stressful than that of the aorta. Still, they must handle changes in blood pressure, so they also are constructed of tough, heavy-duty elastic material. They are not nearly as large as regular arteries. Arterioles are about as thin as a piece of dental floss.

MOVING TOWARD THE HEART

Veins have a multilayered structure similar to arteries, but their walls are thinner. They also do not have the elastic, rubber-band abilities that arteries possess. Just as a water hose does not usually have bulges in sections, arteries can maintain the same shape no matter how much blood is pushed through them. Veins can vary their shape, going from flat to fat, depending on the amount of blood pressure. It is even possible to see this by raising a hand above the level of the heart. Veins on the back of the hand thin

Tunica interna

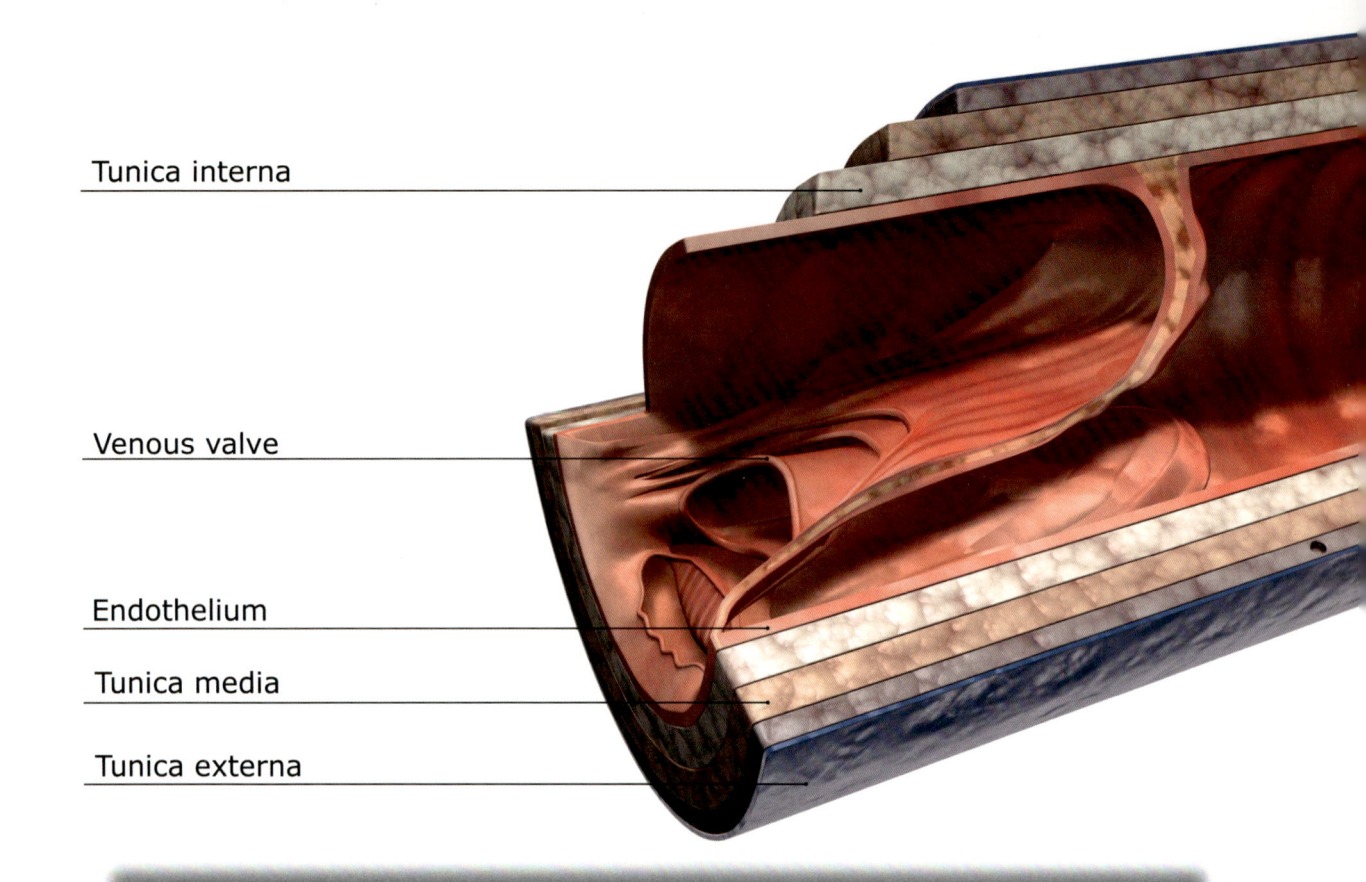

Venous valve

Endothelium

Tunica media

Tunica externa

This image shows the parts of a vein wall, as well as a valve. The insides of blood vessels are lined with epithelial tissue, which can also be found in the endocardium.

out as blood pressure slows. When the hand is placed below the heart, the veins bulge slightly as the pressure increases.

Inside every vein is a valve. Similar to the valves in the heart, these structures help to ensure that blood flows in one direction. Instead of the parachute-like form of heart valves, vein valves look a bit like a letter "w" with a slit in the middle. As the muscles in the walls of veins move with blood pressure, the valve opens or closes to maintain an even flow.

Large veins, like the pulmonary vein, are about 1 inch (2.5 cm) thick. Smaller veins are only about as thick as a fine strand of hair. The smallest veins are called venules. These miniscule veins begin at the capillaries.

CONNECTING VEINS AND ARTERIES

Capillaries form an almost invisible link between the veins and arteries. That is because capillaries are extremely small. Their walls are only one cell thick. If twenty-five capillaries were stacked in a pile end to end, they would measure 1 inch (2.5 cm). Despite their small size, capillaries make up 99 percent of the entire circulatory system. Every individual has about 10 billion capillaries.

Returning to the mail delivery analogy, capillaries are like the mailman who delivers a package directly to a household. In this case, the package consists of food and oxygen and the recipient is a single cell. Capillaries also pick up wastes and other unwanted products from cells.

During the exchange process, individual red blood cells squeeze through the tiny capillaries in a single file to reach body cells. Amazingly, the process occurs within one to three seconds, and then the red blood cells leave the capillaries and return to the veins.

While capillaries are hard to see with the naked eye, their presence can become visible through skin color changes. For example, a person who is blushing has increased blood flow

THE HEART IN 3D

to the facial capillaries. Stretching the skin around the mouth to make a funny face turns surrounding skin a lighter color, as blood flow in the capillaries decreases.

Tiny air sacs in the lungs, called alveoli, are the sites where blood absorb oxygen and releases carbon dioxide. The alveoli are covered with a dens network of capillaries.

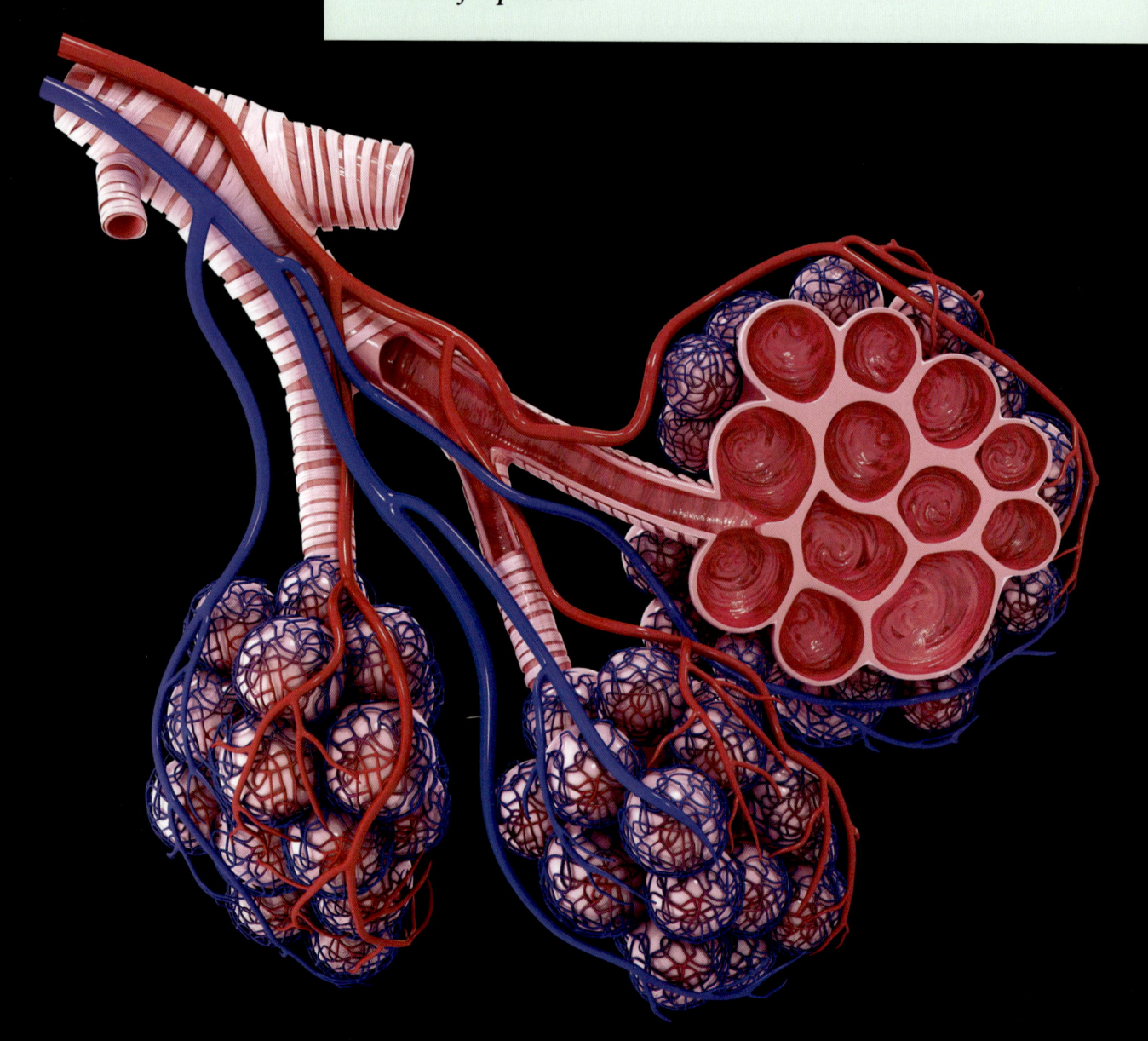

CIRCULATION

To circulate means to move along a path until you come back to a starting point, from which the whole process continuously repeats. In terms of blood, circulation refers to its movement from and to the heart through the arteries and veins. The heart is like a crossroads, where all smaller roads end up. Like cars on a miniature racetrack, blood cells speed through arteries and veins. A drop of oxygen-rich blood begins its journey from the heart to the right fingertips by being squeezed out of the heart's left ventricle. It zooms through the aorta with incredible speed.

The blood then travels across the shoulder through the subclavian artery. Similar to a fork in the road, this artery

WHAT CAUSES BRUISES?

Everybody at some point gets a bruise after falling off a skateboard, getting hit by a baseball, or experiencing some other accident that causes capillaries near the skin's surface to break. At first a bruise looks reddish, due to the oxygen-rich hemoglobin in the red blood cells that leaks out of the broken capillaries.

After a few hours, the hemoglobin begins to break down and the bruise becomes bluish or purplish in color. As the bruise begins to heal, it turns greenish and then yellowish. This is due to the presence of chemicals that are the result of the breakdown of hemoglobin.

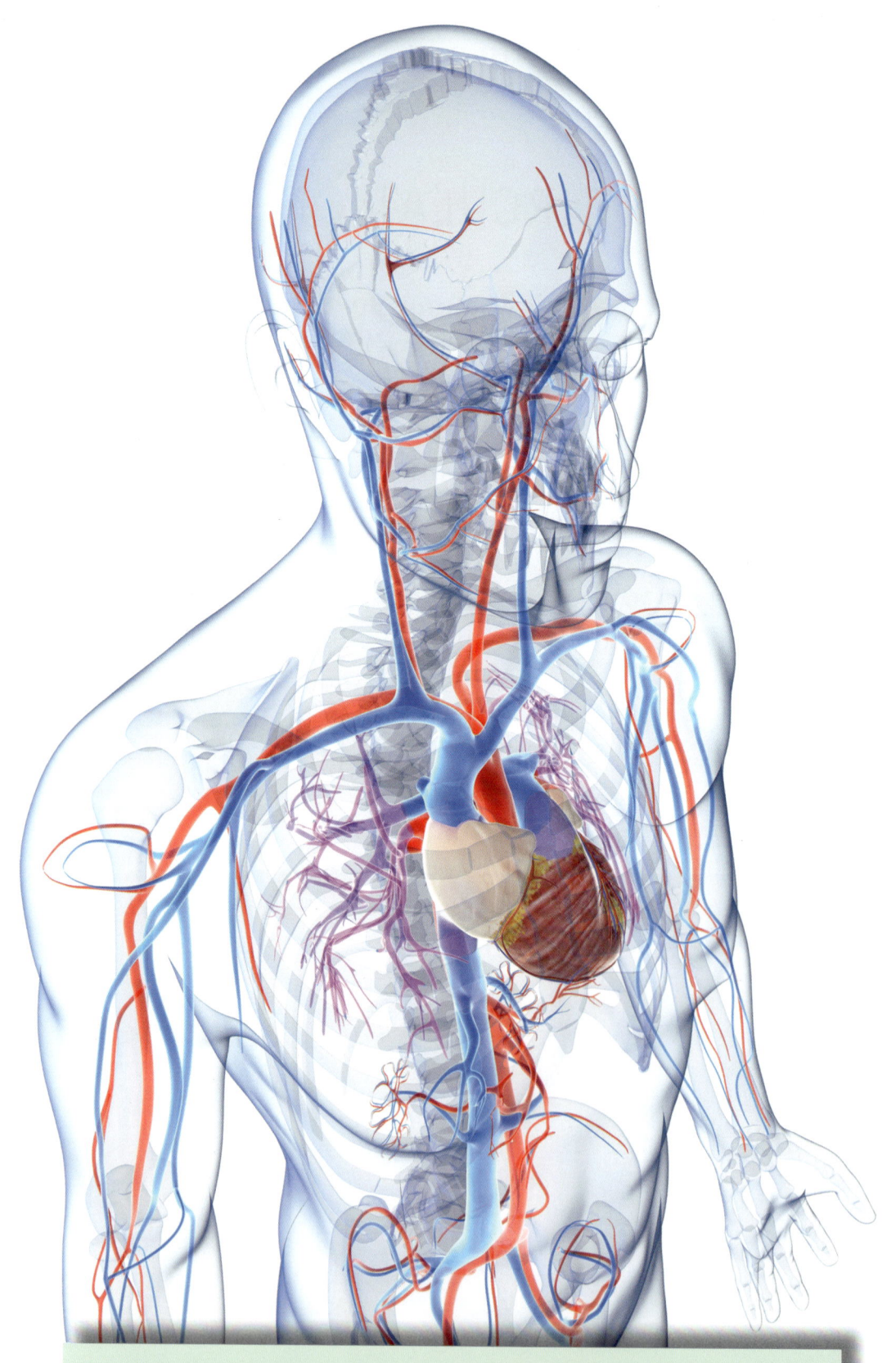

To reach the fingertips of the right hand from the heart, blood travels through the aorta, brachiocephalic artery, right subclavian artery, axillary artery, brachial artery, radial or ulnar arteries, palmar arch, and digital arteries.

branches into the thinner brachial artery, which goes down the center of the right arm. There are other possible roads blood can then take, such as the radial artery or the ulnar artery. These arteries run on either side of the arm.

At this point the blood has slowed down to a nice cruising speed, now that it is away from all of the heart's pumping action. In fact, blood in the arm travels about one thousand times slower than blood that has just left the heart and zipped through the aorta. Like sightseers on a road trip, blood does not want to miss anything. It delivers oxygen and nutrients to every part of the arm and also picks up cell wastes. Blood on this route ends up at the digital arteries on the hands' fingertips. As the arteries narrow, they turn into the smaller arterioles and then into miniscule capillaries.

Capillaries gradually become wider and merge into veins. Here is where the vein valves come in handy. Consider that the blood must travel back up the arm, defying gravity. The valves make sure that blood flows in the right direction, instead of puddling up in the hands. The veins merge into a big vein, appropriately called the superior vena cava, which means the upper main vein. It collects all of the blood from the entire upper portion of the body and sends it back to the heart.

A similar trip is taken by blood to the legs, except it travels down different arteries and comes back through different veins. Blood to the right leg, for example, goes through the descending aorta in the center of the body and

THE HEART IN 3D

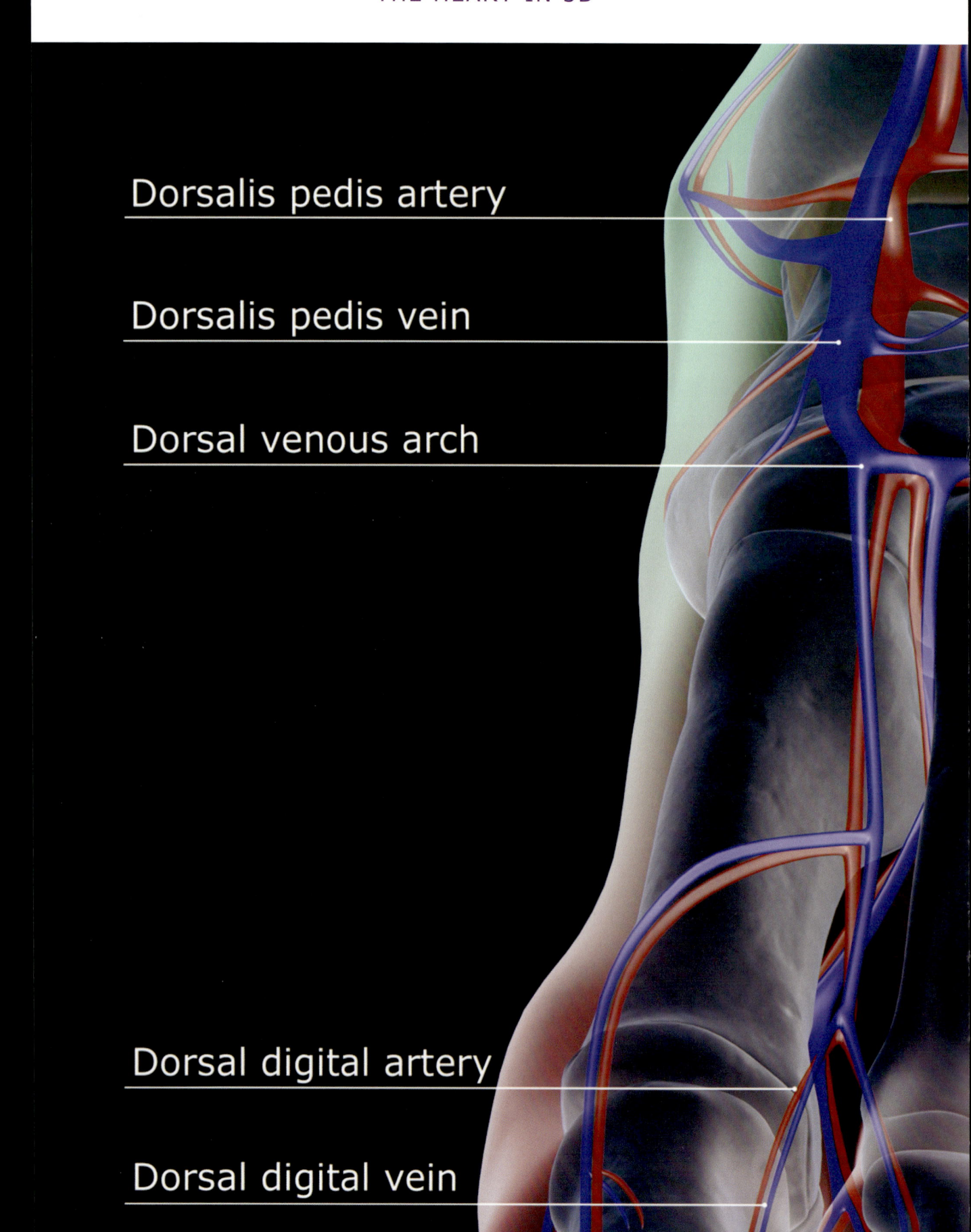

Dorsalis pedis artery

Dorsalis pedis vein

Dorsal venous arch

Dorsal digital artery

Dorsal digital vein

MOVING THROUGH THE SYSTEM

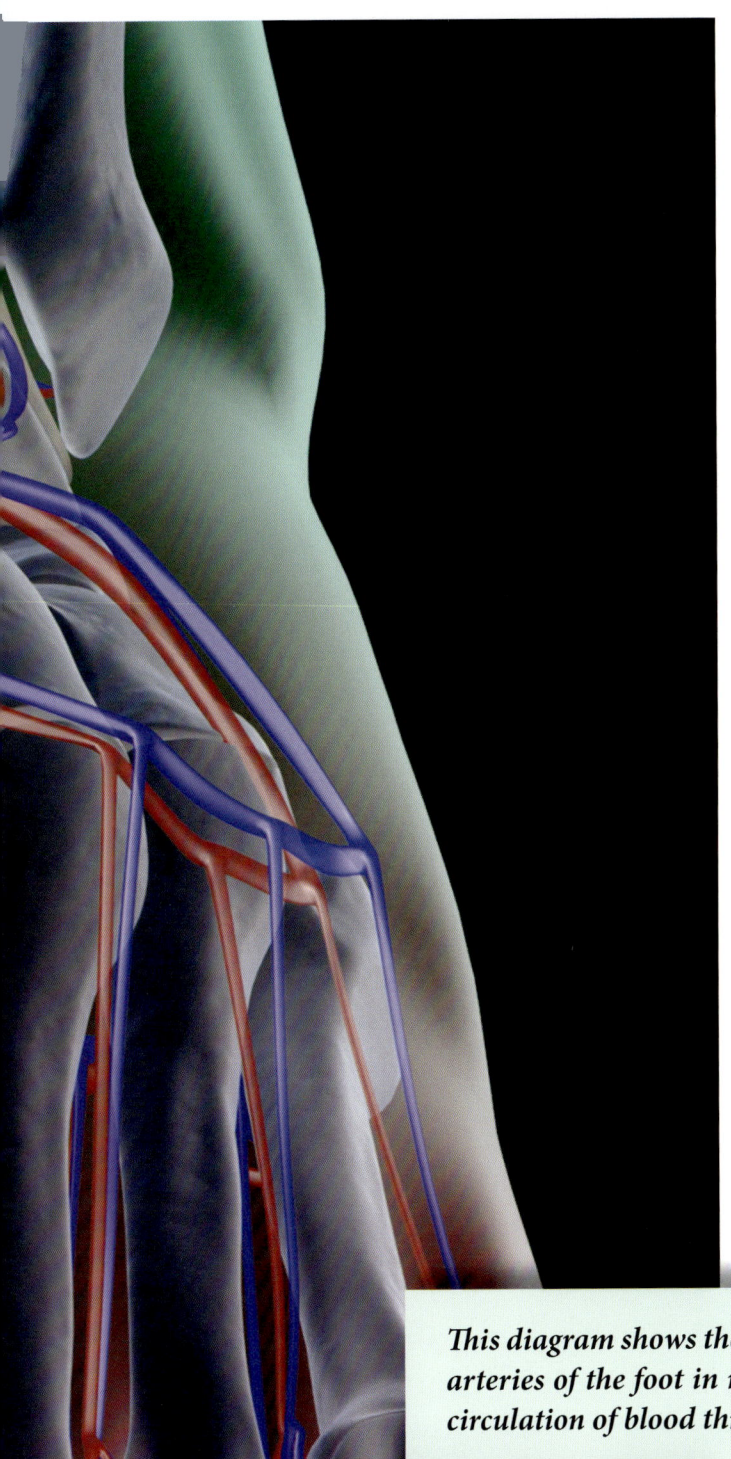

down through a bunch of leg arteries, including the femoral artery, which is a big artery in the middle of the leg. Veins, such as the large femoral vein, send blood back to the heart through the inferior vena cava. Inferior in this case does not mean second rate, but instead refers to the fact that the vein is located below the heart. The inferior vena cava is like the twin of the superior vena cava, except it collects blood from the body's lower half for return to the heart.

This diagram shows the veins of the foot in blue and the arteries of the foot in red. They are responsible for the circulation of blood throughout the foot.

39

CHAPTER FOUR

THE KIDNEYS

The body runs in an impressively efficient manner. However, it does produce waste, or substances that people do not need. The kidneys have the monumental task of cleaning out most of this unnecessary material. Each individual is born with two kidneys, which look like beans or boxing gloves. In between the kidneys are two long tubes. The large one on the left, as you face a body, is the inferior vena cava, the vein that brings blood back to the heart from the lower part of the body. The big tube on the right is the aorta, the super artery that sends blood out through the heart.

The large tubes that connect the kidneys to the aorta are called the main renal arteries. There actually are several renal arteries, ranging from large to small. As most arteries do, they fan out into branches, in this case becoming smaller the closer they get to the kidney.

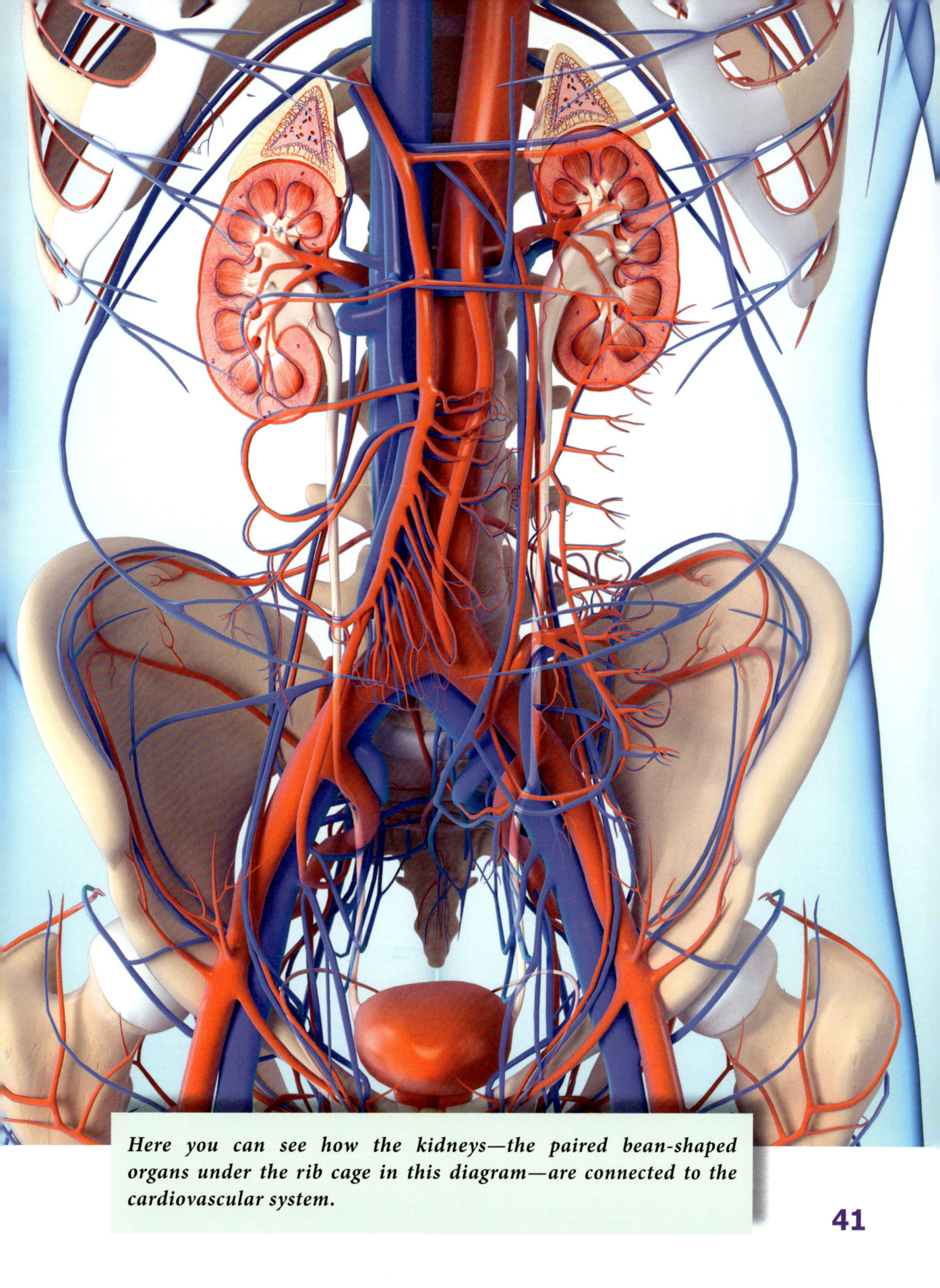

Here you can see how the kidneys—the paired bean-shaped organs under the rib cage in this diagram—are connected to the cardiovascular system.

The outermost part of the kidney, which in side view looks like a human ear, is called the renal capsule. Underneath the renal capsule lies the kidney cortex. It looks like an earflap. This part of the kidney contains very small filters called nephrons that separate waste matter from blood.

THE NEPHRONS

Each kidney has over a million nephrons. Nephrons function like microscopic coffee filters, allowing blood to flow through them like water so that a person ends up with waste material that can be discarded and cleaned blood that can be circulated back through the body. Nephrons are found in kidney tissues called renal pyramids, which really do look a bit like pyramids. The nephron microfilters consist of three main parts: renal corpuscles, tubules, and blood vessels.

Together, the glomerulus and the Bowman's capsule make up a renal corpuscle. The glomerulus is a tangled knot of capillaries. The Bowman's capsule is the structure that surrounds it. Blood from an arteriole flows into the renal corpuscle. Water from that blood can pass through the walls of the glomerulus. So can wastes—like excess salt and sugar—that are dissolved in it. Essential blood cells and proteins, however, cannot pass through. The glomerular walls act as a kind of strainer that prevent larger sized objects, which in this case are the essential components of blood, from seeping through. The filtered blood then flows out through another arteriole.

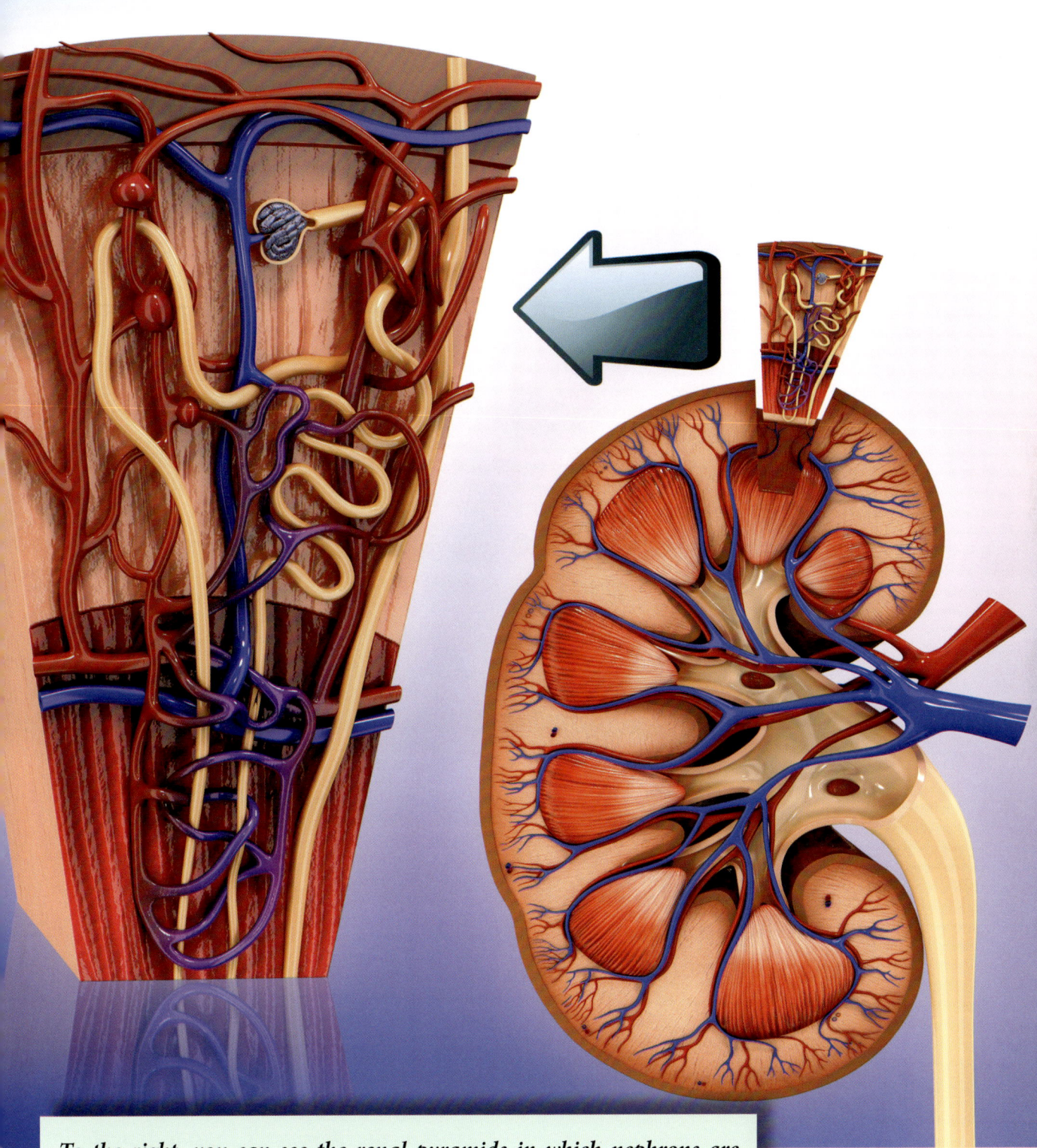

To the right, you can see the renal pyramids in which nephrons are located. The detail to the left shows a nephron, with its blood vessels, tubules, and renal corpuscle.

43

THE HEART IN 3D

At any time during the day, the glomerulus capillaries contain about 4.6 fluid ounces (.13 liter) of blood. Each day, these tiny filters remove approximately 50 gallons (189 l) of fluid from blood. That would be like trying to separate the water from the solids out of fifty large containers of milk. Just as the human heart is one of the world's finest pumps, the kidneys contain some of the world's best filters. Even the most high-tech coffee or car filter pales in comparison with the job the kidneys perform each day.

The liquid that is filtered out by the glomerulus is carried away through small pipes called tubules. A network

The glomerulus is made up of a bundle of capillaries. Its role is to filter water and wastes out of the blood. It is enclosed within the Bowman's capsule (purple in this diagram).

of blood vessels wraps around the twisting loops these tubules make. Here, in a second filtration process, most of the water and minerals that were previously separated from blood are reabsorbed. Every person needs a certain quantity of water and minerals, and the second filtering removes what the body needs.

The body makes hormones that control the amount of water that is reabsorbed by the blood. The ability to control how much water gets reabsorbed is very useful. For example, after a long, hot summer day full of fun activities a person would need more water

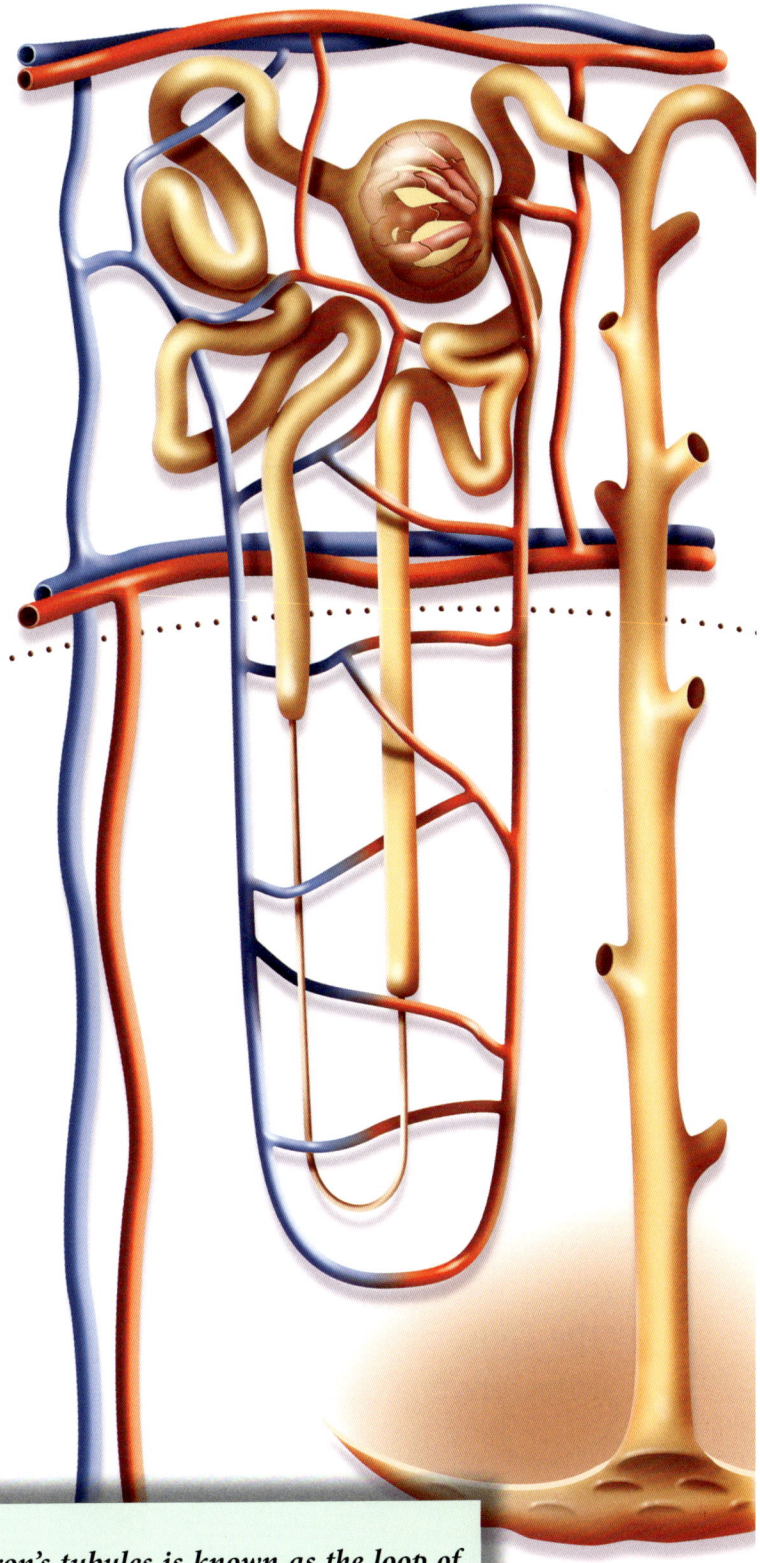

The thin, low loop in a nephron's tubules is known as the loop of Henle, while twisting parts are called the distal and proximal convoluted tubules.

because he or she would likely sweat more, thereby getting rid of more fluids. A person drinking a lot of beverages on a cold day, though, probably would not require a lot of extra water, so the kidneys would allow for more water to be removed, keeping the body in balance.

Hormones also control the absorption levels of minerals, like calcium and salt. Calcium comes from foods such as dairy products and certain vegetables. It forms the building blocks of bones and teeth. Salt affects blood pressure.

AFTER THE KIDNEYS

After excess water and waste have gone through the second filtration step, the remaining liquid becomes concentrated with undesirable substances like salt, proteins, and acids not needed by the body. This concentrated liquid is called urine. Urine moves down pipes, known as ureters, which lead to the bladder. Urine is held in the bladder until it becomes full. At that point the waste is released from the body through another tube, the urethra.

Once filtered, blood is removed from the kidneys by the renal veins. The veins carry the cleaned blood back through the chest area and into the heart. The left renal vein is longer than the right one. This is because the right kidney is closer to the inferior vena cava.

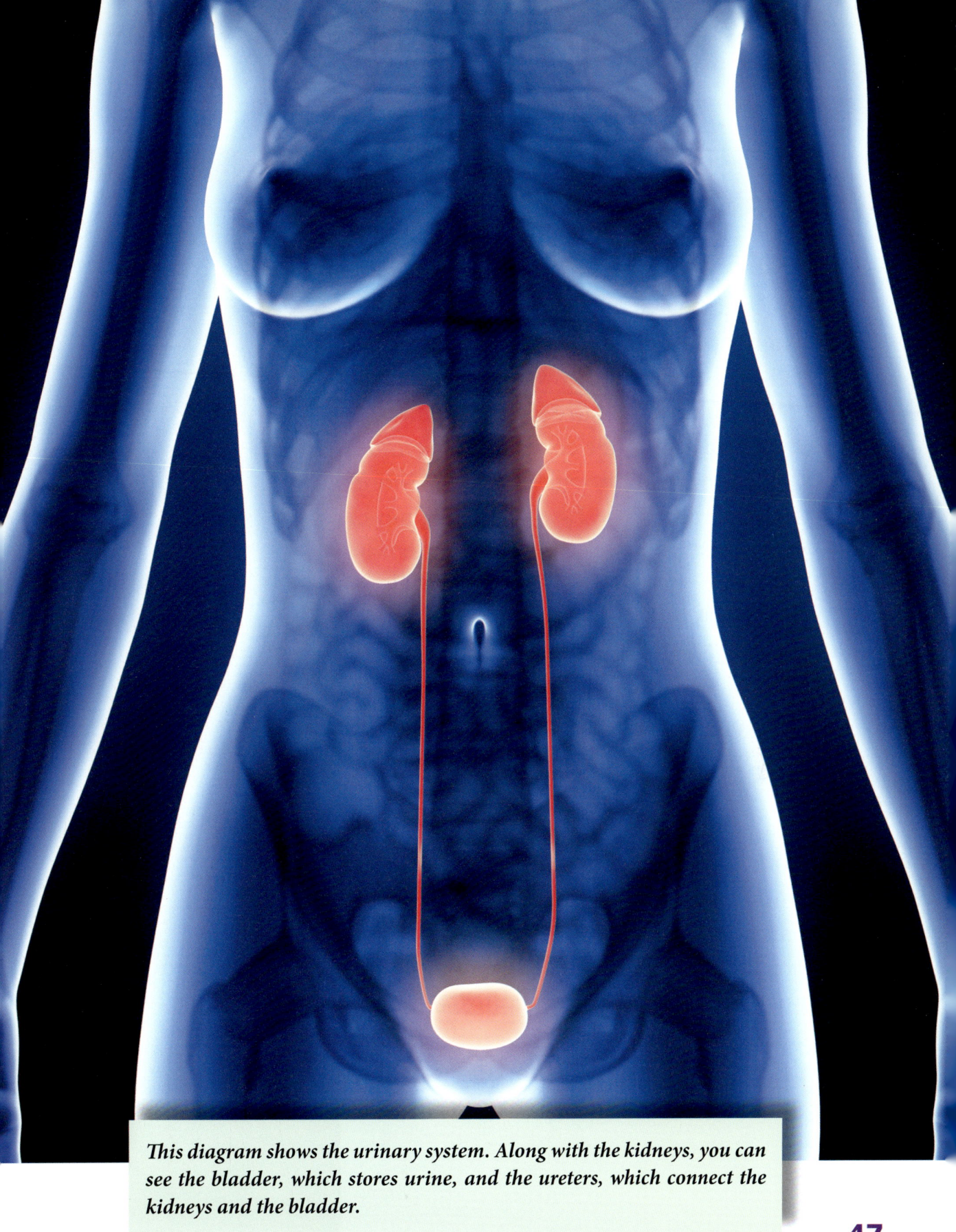

This diagram shows the urinary system. Along with the kidneys, you can see the bladder, which stores urine, and the ureters, which connect the kidneys and the bladder.

47

THE KIDNEYS AND BLOOD PRESSURE

The heart itself creates blood pressure when it pumps blood through the blood vessels. The kidneys, however, also help to control blood pressure. On the simplest level, imagine coffee containing grounds being poured through a filter. More grounds, or, in the case of the kidneys, more waste matter, makes it harder for water to travel through the filter. When this happens, the kidneys produce a chemical known as renin, which helps to create the hormone angiotensin. This hormone raises blood pressure.

Imagine what happens when a person eats a high-sodium meal, like a salty pizza or a hamburger and fries from a fast food restaurant. The high amount of salt causes the kidneys to make a lot of renin, which in turn produces angiotensin. This hormone not only raises blood pressure, but also causes the arteries to narrow. Blood then has a harder time moving through the arteries. The kidneys can also retain

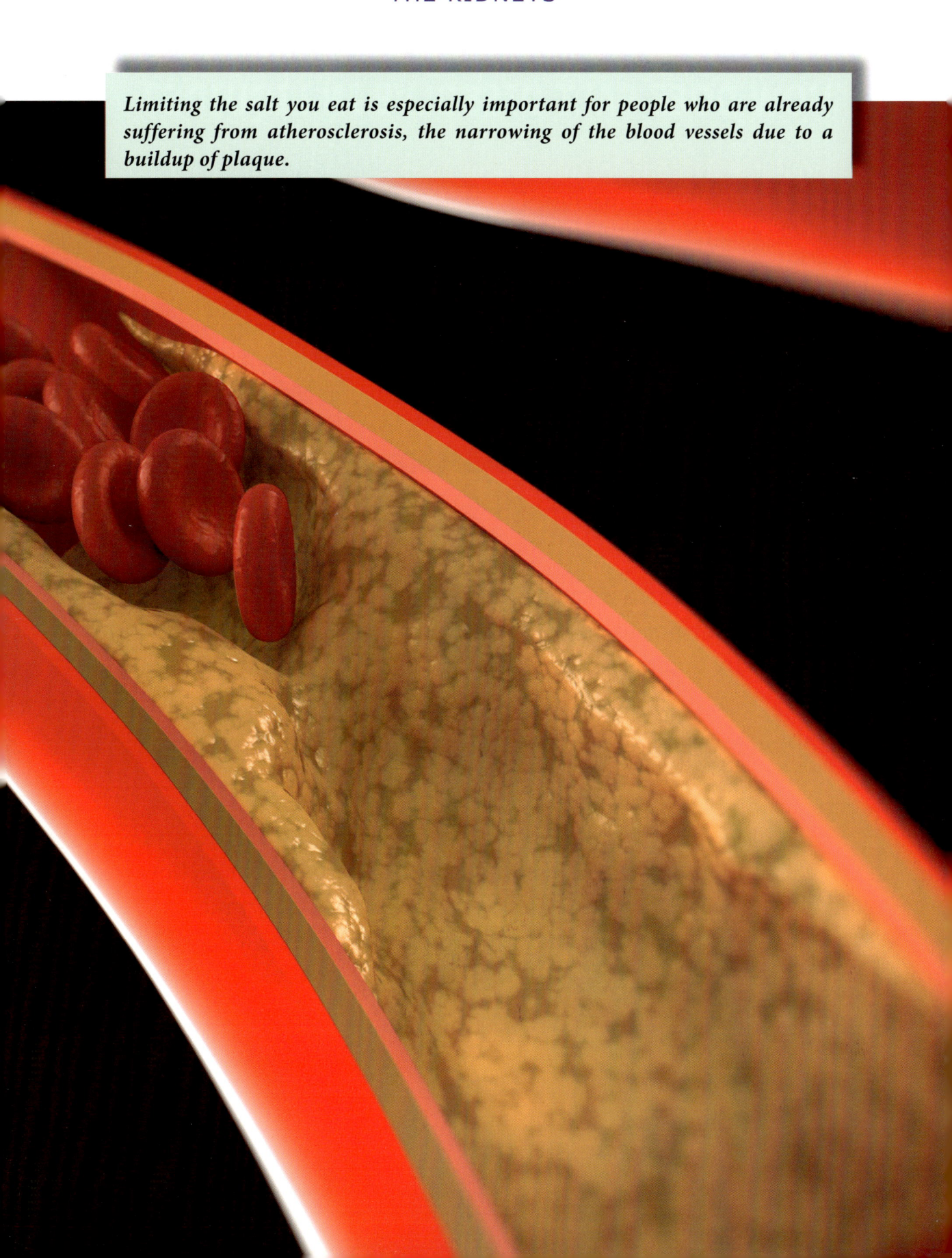

THE KIDNEYS

Limiting the salt you eat is especially important for people who are already suffering from atherosclerosis, the narrowing of the blood vessels due to a buildup of plaque.

HOW DOES SALT DISSOLVE IN LIQUIDS?

Liquids may contain substances in dissolved form, meaning that the materials are broken down into invisible parts. This occurs on a daily basis in urine, the liquid waste produced by kidneys.

To see for yourself how substances such as salt dissolve in water, try mixing a tablespoon of salt into a container full of warm water. Stir the salt until it disappears. Pour some of the mixture onto a clear dish. Allow the dish to sit in a warm place until the water evaporates. The result indicates how dissolved materials can become concentrated in water.

salt, which further causes blood pressure to rise. It is, therefore, important not to consume too much salt to avoid high blood pressure and other health problems.

BLOOD AND YOUR HEALTH

Doctors check to make sure patients have working kidneys and healthy blood. There are a number of tests to check how the kidneys are working. A urinalysis measures how much protein is in a person's urine. High blood pressure can be a sign that the kidneys are not working right. There are several blood tests for kidney disease, too.

To do a blood test, a doctor will take a sample of blood from veins in the arm. Doctors can drop the blood into a container and send it to the laboratory for testing. Scientists may then analyze the blood to determine its contents. Usually a routine blood test involves counting the basic components of blood: red cells, hemoglobin, white cells, and platelets. This is called a blood count. Each number is compared with a standard to check for deficiencies or excesses within the blood. If a person is healthy and the kidneys are in perfect working order, the patient will receive a clean bill of health.

GLOSSARY

ARTERIOLE A small artery.

ARTERY A thick, elastic blood vessel that carries blood away from the heart.

ATRIUM The upper chamber, or enclosed space, found on each side of the heart.

BLADDER A sac that collects urine produced by the kidneys.

BLOOD A liquid that transports oxygen, nutrients, minerals, and hormones to cells in the body. Blood also collects cell wastes, such as carbon dioxide and excess salt, for disposal.

BLOOD VESSEL A tube through which blood moves around the body.

CAPILLARY A very small blood vessel that directly delivers nutrients and oxygen from blood to cells within the body. Capillaries also take in wastes from cells.

CARDIOVASCULAR SYSTEM Consisting of the heart and blood vessels, the cardiovascular system is responsible for circulating, or moving, blood around the body.

CHOLESTEROL A waxy substance found in the bodies of people and other animals.

CLOT To stick together and become hard.

DIABETES An illness in which the body cannot control how much sugar the blood contains. It is caused by a lack of

GLOSSARY

insulin, a substance made by the body that is used to turn sugar into energy.

GLOMERULUS A tangled knot of small blood capillaries in the nephron that helps to filter blood.

HEMOGLOBIN A protein in red blood cells that, when combined with oxygen, turns red. It gives color to blood.

HORMONE A chemical made by the body that controls organ function.

LYMPHOCYTE A kind of white blood cell; lymphocytes fight off infection.

NEPHRON A microscopic filter in the kidneys that cleans blood.

NUTRIENT A substance that an animal or plant needs to continue living.

ORGAN A primary structural part of the body, such as the heart or kidneys, that has an important role to play.

OXYGEN An odorless, invisible gas that energizes cells and is essential to human respiration, or breathing.

PLATELET A doughnut-shaped blood cell that lets blood clot, or stick together and harden, enabling cuts to heal and helping prevent too much blood from leaking out of wounds.

RED BLOOD CELL The kind of blood cell that transports oxygen.

RENIN Made by the kidneys, renin activates production of angiotensin, a hormone in blood that raises blood pressure.

T CELL A lymphocyte that protects the body by killing germs, attacking cancer cells, and controlling hormone levels.

VALVE A device that controls the flow of something, usually a liquid. The heart and veins have valves to control blood flow and to ensure that blood travels in a certain direction.

VEIN A blood vessel that carries blood to the heart from other parts of the body.

VENTRICLE The lower chamber, or enclosed space, found on each side of the heart.

VENULE A small vein.

FOR MORE INFORMATION

American Heart Association

7272 Greenville Avenue

Dallas, TX 75231

(800) 242-8721

Website: http://www.heart.org

This organization, founded by cardiologists in 1924, educates the public about matters relating to the heart and funds research to prevent heart disease and stroke.

Canadian Congenital Heart Alliance

C4-233 Cross Avenue, P.O. Box 233

Oakville, ON L6J 2W9

Canada

Website: http://www.cchaforlife.org

CCHA's mission is to raise awareness about congenital heart conditions among the Canadian public and to support Canadians who are suffering from such conditions. It works with and advocates for both children and adults with congenital heart defects.

Centers for Disease Control and Prevention

Division for Heart Disease and Stroke Prevention

4770 Buford Highway NE, Mail Stop F-72

Atlanta, GA 30341

(800) 232-4636

Website: http://www.cdc.gov/heartdisease

The Heart Disease and Stroke Prevention division of this federal agency issues recommendations for heart health, supplies information about heart disease and strokes, and supports a variety of public health efforts that address heart disease.

Children's Heart Institute—Leesburg

19465 Deerfield Avenue, Suite 310

Leesburg, VA 20176

(571) 291-9025

Website: http://www.childrensheartinstitute.org

These pediatric cardiology facilities for young people also provide educational information about heart disease and how the heart works.

The Franklin Institute

222 North 20th Street

Philadelphia, PA 19103

(215) 448-1200

Website: https://www.fi.edu

The museum and science education center was founded in 1824 and named after Benjamin Franklin, one of the first American scientists. One of its main attractions is a giant model of a human heart that visitors can walk through.

FOR MORE INFORMATION

Heart and Stroke Foundation of Canada
222 Queen Street, Suite 1402
Ottawa, ON K1P 5V9
Canada
(613) 569-4361
Website: http://www.heartandstroke.com

This group aims to prevent disease, save lives, and promote recovery. It educates Canadians on healthy lifestyles, funds research, and works for health equity.

Miller Family Heart & Vascular Institute
Cleveland Clinic Main Campus
9500 Euclid Avenue
Cleveland, OH 44195
(800) 659-7822
Website: https://my.clevelandclinic.org/services/heart

The Cleveland Clinic's prestigious cardiovascular institute is an academic medical center that performs thousands of procedures each year. Its website offers information about the heart and cardiovascular problems.

WomenHeart: The National Coalition for Women with Heart Disease
1100 17th Street NW, Suite 500
Washington, DC 20036
(202) 728-7199

Website: http://www.womenheart.org

Founded in 1999 to help women living with or at risk for heart disease, WomenHeart has more than one hundred patient support groups across the United States. Dedicated to education, the group has trained hundreds of women as community educators.

WEBSITES

Because of the changing nature of Internet links, Rosen Publishing has developed an online list of websites related to the subject of this book. This site is updated regularly. Please use this link to access the list:

http://www.rosenlinks.com/HB3D/Heart

FOR FURTHER READING

Amidon, Stephen, and Thomas Amidon. *The Sublime Engine: A Biography of the Human Heart*. Emmaus, PA: Rodale Publishing, 2012.

Ballard, Carol. *Heart and Blood* (Body Focus). 2nd edition. Portsmouth, NH: Heinemann, 2009.

Burstein, John. *The Amazing Circulatory System: How Does My Heart Work?* (Slim Goodbody's Body Buddies). St. Catharines, ON: Crabtree Publishing, 2009.

Caster, Shannon. *Heart* (Body Systems). New York, NY: PowerKids Press, 2010.

Chizner, Michael. *Clinical Cardiology Made Ridiculously Simple* (Medmaster Ridiculously Simple). 4th edition. Miami, FL: Medmaster, 2014.

Cohen, Todd J. *A Patient's Guide to Heart Rhythm Problems*. Baltimore, MD: Johns Hopkins University Press, 2010.

Corcoran, Mary K. *The Circulatory Story*. Watertown, MA: Charlesbridge, 2010.

Levete, Sarah. *Understanding the Heart, Lungs, and Blood*. New York, NY: Rosen Publishing, 2010.

Levy, Daniel, and Susan Brink. *Change of Heart: Unraveling the Mysteries of Cardiovascular Disease*. New York, NY: Vintage, 2006.

Newquist, HP. *The Book of Blood: From Legends and Leeches to Vampires and Veins*. Boston, MA: Houghton Mifflin Harcourt Books for Young Readers, 2012.

Norris, Maggie, and Donna Rae Siegfried. *Anatomy and Physiology For Dummies.* 2nd edition. New York, NY: Wiley, 2011.

Rose, Simon. *The Cardiovascular System* (How the Human Body Works). New York, NY: Weigl Publishers Inc., 2014.

Simon, Seymour. *The Heart: All About Our Circulatory System and More!* New York, NY: Harper Collins, 2006.

Storad, Conrad J. *Your Circulatory System* (Searchlight Books: How Does Your Body Work?). Minneapolis, MN: LernerClassroom, 2012.

INDEX

A
albumin, 20–22
anemia, 20
angina, 5
angioplasty, 8
angiotensin, 48
antigens, 24
aorta, 12–13, 31, 35, 37, 40
aortic valve, 15, 17
arrhythmias, 5
arteries, 7, 11, 12, 13, 18, 28, 29–31, 33, 35–39, 40, 48
arterioles, 31, 37, 42
atherosclerosis, 5, 7
atriums, 13, 17

B
B cells, 25
bladder, 46
blood
    about, 4, 18–27
    clotting of, 5, 27
    components of, 20
blood cells, 5
blood pressure, 7, 31, 32, 46, 48–50
blood test, 51
blood type, 24
blood vessels, 5, 8, 28, 45, 48
Bowman's capsule, 42
    brachial artery, 37
bruises, 35

C
capillaries, 33–34, 35, 37, 42, 44
carbon dioxide, 4, 13, 22
cardiac vein, 11
cardiomyopathy, 5
cardiovascular system, 4, 28
    problems with, 5–8
centrifuge, 20
cholesterol, 5, 7
chordae tendineae, 13–15
circulation, 35–39
coronary arteries, 11
coronary bypass surgery, 7

D
diabetes, 7
diet, 7, 20, 46, 48, 50

F
femoral artery, 39
femoral vein, 39

61

G
globulin, 20, 22
glomerulus, 42, 44

H
heart
> about, 4–5, 9–17
> heartbeat/rhythm of, 15–17
> keeping it healthy, 7
> valves, 5, 13–15, 17, 32

heart attack, 5
heartbeat, stages of, 17
heart disease, 5
heart failure, 5
heart murmur, 5
heart rate, 15
heart transplant surgery, 8
hemoglobin, 22, 35, 51
hormones, 20, 45–46, 48

I
infections, fighting, 24–25
inferior vena cava, 39, 40, 46
iron, 20

K
kidney cortex, 42
kidneys, 4, 40–50

L
liver, 20, 28
lumen, 31

lungs, 4, 13, 15, 17, 22, 28, 29
lymphocytes, 24–25

M
marrow, 22, 24
mitral valve, 13
myocardium, 11

N
nephrons, 42

O
oxygen, 4, 5, 11, 13, 17, 18, 22, 28, 29, 33, 35, 37

P
pacemakers, 8
pericardium, 9
pH, 5
plaque, 5, 8
plasma, 20
platelets, 5, 27, 51
pulmonary artery, 13, 15
pulmonary vein, 13, 29, 32

R
radial artery, 37
red blood cells, 5, 20, 22, 24, 33, 35, 51
renal arteries, 40
renal capsule, 42
renal corpuscle, 42
renal pyramids, 42
renin, 48

INDEX

S
stroke, 5
subclavian artery, 35–37
superior vena cava, 37, 39

T
T cells, 25
tricuspid valve, 13, 15
tubules, 44–45

U
ulnar artery, 37
urethra, 46

urinalysis, 50
urine, 46, 50

V
veins, 11, 12, 13, 28–29, 31–33, 35, 37, 39, 40, 46, 51
    valves, 32, 37
ventricles, 13, 15, 17, 35
venules, 33

W
wastes, 4, 22, 33, 37, 40, 42, 48, 50
white blood cells, 5, 20, 24, 51

ABOUT THE AUTHORS

Anna Kingston has written several books for elementary school readers, including *The Life Cycle of a Sea Turtle* and *The Life Cycle of a Pelican*. A native of New Jersey, she now lives on Long Island.

Jennifer Viegas is a reporter for Discovery Channel Online News and is a features columnist for Knight Ridder newspapers. She has worked as a journalist for ABC News, PBS, the *Washington Post*, the *Christian Science Monitor*, and other media. Jennifer also helped to write two heart-healthy cookbooks for *Cooking Light*.

PHOTO CREDITS

Cover, p. 1 (heart) Sebastian Kaulitzki/Shutterstock.com; cover, p. 1 (hand) © iStockphoto.com/Nixxphotography; p. 4 sankalpmaya/iStock/Thinkstock; pp. 6, 30 SCIEPRO/Science Photo Library/Getty Images; pp. 7, 26, 44, 45 BSIP/UIG/Getty Images; p. 9 Phanie/Science Source; p. 10 Stocktrek Images/Getty Images; pp. 12, 41 MediaForMedical/UIG/Getty Images; p. 14 Medi-mation/Science Photo Library/Getty Images; p. 16 Marc Phares/Science Source/Getty Images; pp. 19, 34, 43 Pixologicstudio/Science Photo Library/Getty Images; p. 21 Nerthuz/iStock/Thinkstock; pp. 22–23 Reshavskyi/Shutterstock.com; p. 25 Juan Gartner/Science Photo Library/Getty Images; pp. 29, 36, 47 Sebastian Kaulitzki/Science Photo Library/Getty Images; pp. 32, 38–39 MedicalRF.com/Getty Images; pp. 48–49 Science Photo Library – SCIEPRO/Brand X Pictures/Getty Images; back cover (figure) © iStockphoto.com/comotion design; cover and interior pages graphic elements © iStockphoto.com/StudioM1, wenani/Shutterstock.com, Egor Tetiushev/Shutterstock.com.

Designer: Brian Garvey; Editor: Amelie von Zumbusch;
Photo Researcher: Karen Huang

5/4/16